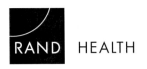

Transforming Systems for Parental Depression and Early Childhood Developmental Delays

Findings and Lessons Learned from the *Helping Families Raise Healthy Children* Initiative

Dana Schultz, Kerry A. Reynolds, Lisa M. Sontag-Padilla, Susan L. Lovejoy, Ray Firth, Harold Alan Pincus

Prepared for the Community Care Behavioral Health Organization

The research described in this report was prepared for the Community Care Behavioral Health Organization and was conducted within RAND Health, a division of the RAND Corporation.

Library of Congress Cataloging-in-Publication Data is available for this publication.

ISBN: 978-0-8330-7996-1

The RAND Corporation is a nonprofit institution that helps improve policy and decisionmaking through research and analysis. RAND's publications do not necessarily reflect the opinions of its research clients and sponsors.

Cover photo courtesy iStockphoto

RAND® is a registered trademark

Published 2013 by the RAND Corporation
1776 Main Street, P.O. Box 2138, Santa Monica, CA 90407-2138
1200 South Hayes Street, Arlington, VA 22202-5050
4570 Fifth Avenue, Suite 600, Pittsburgh, PA 15213-2665
RAND URL: http://www.rand.org/
To order RAND documents or to obtain additional information, contact
Distribution Services: Telephone: (310) 451-7002;
Fax: (310) 451-6915; Email: order@rand.org

Preface

The *Helping Families Raise Healthy Children* initiative was the fourth phase of the Allegheny County Maternal and Child Health Care Collaborative's efforts to implement changes in the local system of maternal and child health care. The initiative targeted three components of service delivery:

1. screening and identification of at-risk families through three pathways within and between the Part C early intervention system and the maternal and child health care system
2. referrals for those identified as being at risk
3. engagement in relationship-based services in both the Part C early intervention and behavioral health systems.

The RAND Corporation conducted the evaluation of the *Helping Families Raise Healthy Children* initiative in collaboration with two other organizing partners, Community Care Behavioral Health and The Alliance for Infants and Toddlers. Community Care Behavioral Health is a nonprofit behavioral health managed care organization founded by the University of Pittsburgh Medical Center that manages the delivery of behavioral health services in the Northeastern part of the United States. Its mission is to improve the health and well-being of the community through the delivery of effective, cost-efficient, and accessible behavioral health services, and its network comprises more than 1,600 service providers and 1.5 million members. The Alliance for Infants and Toddlers, Inc., was established in 1988 by a federal grant to assist families of infants with low birth weights. In 1992, The Alliance became the early intervention service coordination agency for families with concerns about their child's development, handling children from birth to the age of three years. The Alliance conducts developmental assessments and provides a broad array of services and support to children with identified delays.

The evaluation plan encompassed a mixed-methods approach to evaluate the initiative, using three types of measures that employ both quantitative and qualitative data. Process measures helped determine the extent to which the initiative components were being implemented according to plan. System impact measures at the provider and family level offered perspectives on implementation and system changes. Individual outcome measures were assessed at the caregiver level and indicated whether the implementation components were associated with decreases in depressive symptoms and parenting stress and with improvements in caregiver and child health. This document provides the results of the evaluation and will be of interest to policymakers, community leaders, health care providers, and others interested in improvements in the maternal and child health care system.

We would like to thank the members of our Family Advisory Council, who provided valuable insights and feedback for the planning and implementation of the initiative. We would also like to thank the many organizations and individuals who contributed to this project, including Achieva, the Allegheny County Department of Human Services (Office of Behavioral Health, Maternal and Child Health Program), Allegheny Family Network, The Birth Circle, The Children's Home of Pittsburgh, Children's Hospital Primary Care Practices, Early Head Start/Council of Three Rivers American Indian Center, Early Intervention Specialists, the Early Learning Institute, Every Child, Family Resources, Family Centers of the Allegheny Intermediate Unit, Family Foundations Early Head Start, Family Services of Western PA, Gateway Health Plan, Healthy Start, Holy Family Institute, Integrated Care, KidsPlus Pediatrics, Matilda Theiss Child Development Center, McKeesport Perinatal Depression Collaborative, Mercy Behavioral Health, Milestone Centers, Mon Yough Community Services, National Fatherhood Initiative, Pediatric Therapy Professionals, Primary Health Care Centers, Inc. (Alma Illery), Re:solve Crisis Network, Sojourner House, Sto Rox Family Health Center, Turtle Creek Valley MH/MR, Unison Health Plan, UPMC Family Medicine, UPMC for You, Wesley Spectrum Services, and Western Pennsylvania School for the Deaf.

The *Helping Families Raise Healthy Children* initiative and this work were supported by the Robert Wood Johnson Foundation Local Funding Partnership grant program, the Highmark Foundation as the nominating funder, and other local funding partners: UPMC Health Plan, The Pittsburgh Foundation, The Fine Foundation, FISA Foundation, and the Jewish Healthcare Foundation, with additional support from the Allegheny County Department of Human Services, Office of Behavioral Health, and the Pennsylvania Department of Public Welfare. The research was conducted within RAND Health, a division of the RAND Corporation. The RAND Health Quality Assurance process employs peer reviewers, including at least one reviewer who is external to the RAND Corporation. This study benefited from the rigorous technical reviews of Brad Stein and Robert Gallen, which served to improve the quality of this report. A profile of RAND Health, abstracts of its publications, and ordering information can be found at www.rand.org/health.

Contents

Figures

Tables

Summary

The *Helping Families Raise Healthy Children* Initiative

Depression affects millions of Americans each year and is much more likely to affect women. Among low-income and other underserved populations (e.g., minority women), the estimated prevalence rates for maternal depression ranges from 25 to 35 percent (Lanzi et al., 1999; Miranda and Green, 1999; Onunaku, 2005; Siefert et al., 2000). This is markedly higher than depression rates of the general population, which are around 12 percent for women (Narrow, 1998). Untreated maternal depression has potentially serious consequences for a woman's overall well-being, her functioning as a mother, the family's functioning, and her child's development (Onunaku, 2005; Field, 2000). Further, parental depression and the risk of childhood developmental problems often co-occur. Children of depressed parents experience more social and emotional problems than children whose mothers are not depressed, and these children may also experience delays or impairments in cognitive and linguistic development and social interactions. In addition, children of parents with chronic depression are more likely to develop long-term behavioral problems and are at greater risk of behavioral and emotional problems later in life, including depression, anxiety, and conduct disorders. In turn, a child's developmental delays can heighten parental stress, ultimately increasing the risk for parental depression and perpetuating a cycle that affects both parent and child.

Despite the close connection between parental depression and childhood developmental risks, the systems that treat these problems rarely intersect. Part C of the Federal Individuals with Disabilities Education Act (IDEA) provides for a federal grant program that assists states in operating comprehensive early intervention programs for children ages 0–3 with disabilities. Thus, the early intervention system for children at risk of developmental problems is likely to miss opportunities to screen parents for risk of depression—while, conversely, the maternal health care and behavioral health systems treating caregivers with depression are unlikely to identify child development issues that may be increasing family stress and contributing to caregiver depression.

To address this disconnect, a group of partners in the Pittsburgh area involved with the behavioral health, early intervention, and maternal and child health care systems undertook an effort to improve care for families facing the dual challenges of caregiver depression and early childhood developmental delays. This initiative—called *Helping Families Raise Healthy Children*—began in 2009 under the auspices of the Allegheny County Maternal and Child Health Care Collaborative, a broad-based community coalition that has been operating in Pennsylvania since 2002. The initiative's overarching goal was to build a sustainable cross-system infrastructure that improves local capacity to identify and engage families with caregivers experiencing or at risk for depression and children at risk for developmental delays using relationship-based approaches.

To accomplish this goal, the initiative had three specific objectives:

- improve identification of families with primary caregivers at risk for or experiencing depression and infants/toddlers at risk for or experiencing developmental delays
- enhance access to support and services for these families through cross-system referrals for assessment or services in the Medicaid maternal and child health, behavioral health, and early intervention systems
- offer and support engagement in relationship-based services in the early intervention and behavioral health systems that address the needs of both caregivers and young children in the context of the parent-child relationship.

Key Stakeholder Groups

To achieve the initiative's three aims, the Collaborative convened seven stakeholder groups to work together. These groups and their roles and responsibilities relate to the aims of the initiative as follows:

- Families at dual risk for depression and early childhood developmental delays were the target population of the initiative and provided advice during the planning and implementation phases on the initiative implementation protocols, strategies, and materials through a Family Advisory Council.
- Community Care Behavioral Health Organization (Community Care), which is the Medicaid behavioral health managed care organization (MCO), provided care management and ensured access to available resources and services for identified families in an effort to increase the likelihood that they would effectively engage in behavioral health treatment. Community Care provided the organizational and project leadership and facilitated the involvement of the behavioral health network of providers.
- The Alliance for Infants and Toddlers (The Alliance), which is the central intake and service coordination unit for families of children (birth to three years of age), screened and identified families at high risk for depression and took steps to link them to available supports, services, and treatments. The Alliance also educated and supported all service coordinators in a relationship-based approach to service coordination.
- Early intervention service provider organizations (birth to three years of age) provided in-home, relationship-based services for the child's developmental delays.
- Behavioral health provider organizations offered a range of well-established treatments meeting the needs and preferences of referred families with very young children. Community Care developed a network of behavioral health providers able to offer home-based mental health treatment services for families receiving Medicaid.
- Maternal and child health care providers and organizations in the community identified families at high risk for depression and referred them to The Alliance for screening and developmental assessment.
- State and local purchasers and policymakers supported practice and policy changes aimed at enhancing the ability of systems partners to carry out their agreed-upon roles.

Other organizations in the community also offered supports (such as funding, data collection and analysis, and access to requisite resources and services outside the maternal and child health care system) to contribute to successful and sustainable systems change.

This report presents the results of the process, individual outcomes, and system impact measures; offers lessons drawn from a comprehensive evaluation of the program's impact; and concludes with recommendations for practice and policy change designed to expand and sustain the initiative's achievements.

Evaluation Approach

To evaluate the initiative's success in accomplishing its goals, a team from RAND used a mixed-methods approach drawing on both quantitative and qualitative data using three types of measures: process, individual outcome, and system impact (Figure S.1).

Process measures helped determine the extent to which the initiative components were being implemented according to plan, thus providing vital information for potential real-time course corrections. Individual outcome measures indicated whether the implementation components (i.e., screening and identification, referral, and engagement in relationship-based services and treatment) were associated with decreases in depressive symptoms and parenting stress at the caregiver level and with improvements in caregiver and child health. System impact measures at the provider and system levels provided information on the factors affect-

Figure S.1
Process, System Impact, and Outcome Measures

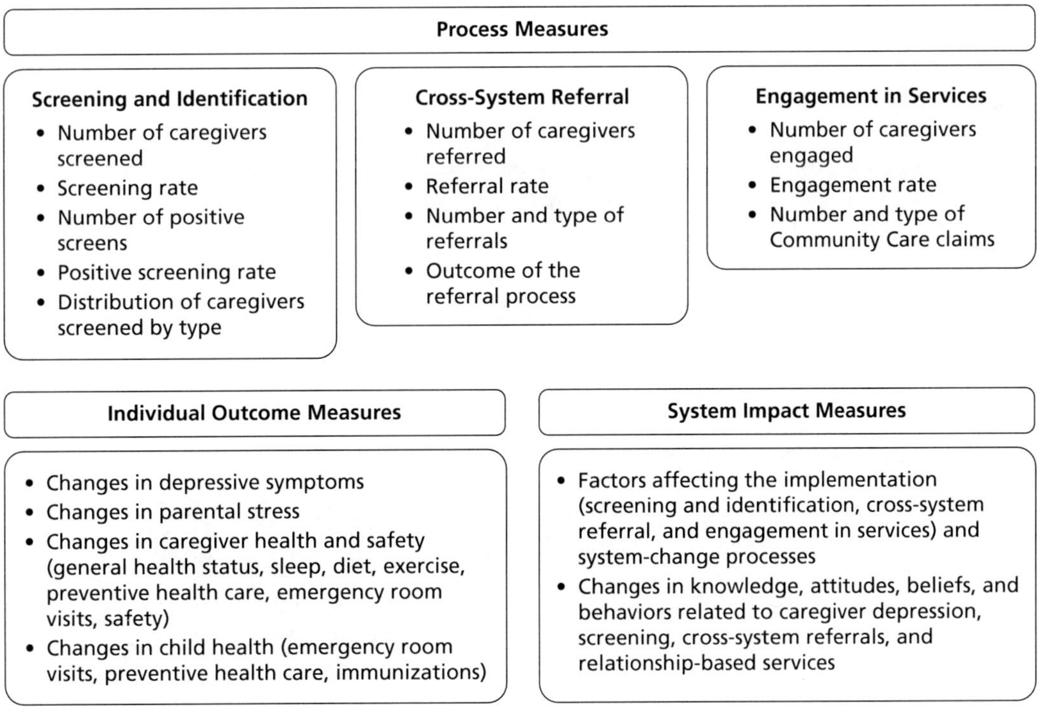

RAND RR122-S.1

ing implementation and improvements in provider knowledge, attitudes, beliefs, and behaviors regarding caregiver depression, infant-caregiver attachment, and relationship-based care.

Evaluation Results

Implementation Process Results

The initiative's implementation strategy was designed to achieve sustainable improvements in processes and outcomes by seeking to

- foster understanding of and response to families' needs and preferences
- establish a cross-system collaborative network
- improve providers' capacity to deliver relationship-based care
- establish cross-system practices and policies for these efforts.

To support these aims, the initiative implemented processes for screening and identifying at-risk families, providing referrals, and supporting engagement in services (Figure S.2).

Screening and Identification

Screening and identification occurred through three pathways:

1. a depression screening process for caregivers involved with early intervention services at The Alliance
2. self-identification by families at The Alliance who did not complete the depression screen or screened negative
3. community partners who recognized families as experiencing or being at risk of depression and referred them to The Alliance.

Figure S.2
Key Components of the Initiative

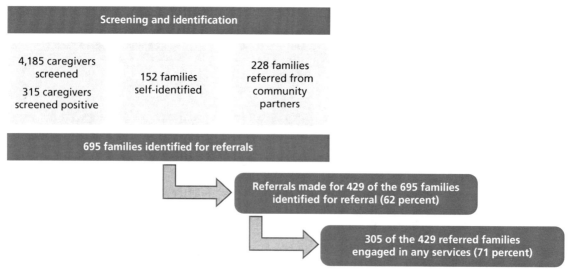

During the 28-month data collection period, service coordinators at The Alliance completed 4,185 depression screens. The overall screening rate for families new to The Alliance was 63 percent, which compares favorably with rates found in descriptive, intervention, and quality improvement studies. Among those screened, 315 caregivers screened positive and were thus identified for the referral component of the initiative. A total of 152 families who did not complete a screening for depression or screened negative self-identified a need for assistance with caregiver depression, and a total of 228 families were identified by community partners as being at risk of caregiver depression and referred to The Alliance for family-centered care, even though their children had not been identified as at risk for developmental delay.

Referral

A total of 695 families were identified for referrals from the three pathways combined: 45 percent from the depression screening at The Alliance, 22 percent from self-identification, and 33 percent via referral from a community partner. Of these 695 families, 429 were referred for services and supports, representing a referral rate of 62 percent. Survey estimates of referral rates following a positive depression screen typically average around 52 percent, although these vary widely according to setting and available follow-up. The initiative's relatively high rate of referral suggests that its cross-system orientation and collaboration, training on referral processes, and additional program supports were effective in helping to ensure that appropriate referrals were made.

Engagement in Services

Of the 429 caregivers referred, 305 engaged in services, for an overall engagement rate of 71 percent. Caregivers were counted as having engaged in services if the family received at least one session of one of the services for which they were referred. For each referred family, The Alliance was able to confirm with the provider whether the family had received any services, but was unable to determine the number of sessions received. This limitation in data collection necessitated a relatively liberal definition of *engagement*, but it is consistent with how other studies define the term (see Table D.3 in Appendix D). This engagement rate was relatively similar across the three different screening and identification pathways: 67 percent for those screened at The Alliance, 75 percent for those self-identified, and 73 percent for those referred by a community-based partner.

Based on comparisons to rates among comparable populations, the engagement rate for the *Healthy Families* initiative was high. Studies of depressed low-income women reported an average baseline engagement rate of approximately 37 percent. One contributing factor to the success of Healthy Families may be the relative ease with which caregivers could obtain services; other factors could include the "warm transfer," in which service coordinators or mental health specialists directly connected caregivers seeking treatment with behavioral health providers; the relationship-based approach that helped caregivers understand the benefits of services for themselves and for their child; and having the referral and connection to services come from a trusted service coordinator.

Figure S.3 summarizes the results of the evaluation of the implementation process.

Figure S.3
Summary of Implementation Process Results (Reference point/initiative)

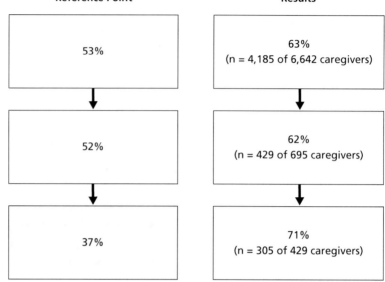

[a] The reference points represent rates found in the literature for similar at-risk populations (e.g., screening: Armstrong and Small, 2007; Garcia, LaCaze, and Ratanasen, 2011; LaRocco-Cockburn et al., 2003; referral: Chaudron et al., 2004; Sheeder, Kabir, and Stafford, 2009; Yonkers et al., 2009; and engagement: Miranda et al., 2003; Smith et al., 2009).

RAND *RR122-S.3*

System Impacts and Factors Affecting Implementation

To assess the initiative's overall impact, we gathered information about changes to the involved Part C early intervention and behavioral health systems as a result of the new processes for three areas: screening and identification of at-risk families, referrals, and engagement in relationship-based services. The system impact measures included changes in knowledge, attitudes, beliefs, and behaviors related to caregiver depression, screening, referrals, and relationship-based services, as well as perspectives from providers and caregivers on the implementation process. We explore the results in the following sections.

Screening and Identification

Appropriate Tools and Protocols for Depression Screening. The consistent screening rate throughout implementation indicates that service coordinators understood and followed the protocol and caregivers accepted the depression screening as a normal part of their interaction with early intervention. This result suggests that with validated tools and well-defined processes, screening for parental depression can be integrated into routine care in the Part C early intervention system.

Training and Ongoing Support for Those Conducting the Screening. Service coordinators and their supervisors reported that being equipped with knowledge, tools, resources, and confidence in their ability to support caregivers is critical to successfully integrating a depression screening protocol into existing processes.

Efforts to Involve the Maternal and Child Health Care System. To engage the maternal and child health care system in making referrals to early intervention based on the caregiver's depression risk, the initiative conducted extensive outreach activities to related community agencies. The results suggest that community-based child and maternal health organizations can take advantage of the system's increased capacity for screening, referral, and treatment services for caregiver depression without overburdening it.

Cross-System Networking and Referrals

Cross-System Networks and Communication Channels. The current systems have evolved in a manner that fosters specialization and fragmentation in treatment and interventions. To improve communication among these systems (thereby cultivating referral and engagement of caregivers in services), the initiative facilitated cross-system trainings and networking meetings that addressed the rationale and importance of referrals and the potential impact on families. Collaborative relationships at every level within and across systems were developed and strengthened through networking meetings, which helped administrators and providers understand each system's role and how to support each other in providing services for at-risk families through cooperative and collaborative efforts. Overall, the efforts to develop cross-system networks and communication channels increased service capacity, communication, and coordination within and between the Part C early intervention and behavioral health systems.

Integration of Referral Processes into Routine Practice. The referral process was developed in conjunction with service coordinators and supervisors. The results suggest that defined protocols and concrete guidance about options enable providers to make knowledgeable and personal referrals that match needs and contribute to a high rate of referral acceptance by families.

"Warm Transfer" Process for Referrals. The referral protocol emphasized directly connecting caregivers to behavioral health services during the early intervention home visit. This "warm transfer" strategy capitalized on the developing relationship and trust between the service coordinator and the caregiver. This type of referral and direct transfer from a trusted provider to other services and supports increased engagement in treatment services.

Coordination and Supports for Referrals. Early intervention programs have historically focused primarily on the child's developmental delays or disabilities in terms of cognition, communication, movement, vision, and hearing. Although social/emotional development has always been an eligible domain for evaluation and treatment in early intervention, needs in this area were generally perceived as the purview of the mental health system. To increase communication and coordination of services across systems, the initiative funded two full-time mental health specialists at The Alliance. These specialists bridged the gap between the behavioral health system and early intervention, which had not previously addressed caregiver depression. Most caregivers found the referral process to be quick and easy and felt that the service coordinator provided the support and encouragement needed to accept and follow through with the referral. However, caregivers also noted a need for improved communication and follow-up after the initial referral. Together, the efforts of the mental health specialists streamlined the referral process and contributed to high referral acceptance rates.

Engagement in Services for At-Risk Families

Capacity-Building Around Relationship-Based Practices. Overall, more than 300 early intervention and behavioral health practitioners working in partner agencies were trained on relationship-based practices. These providers showed increased knowledge about effectively engaging caregivers, infant-caregiver attachment, and relationship-based care. While the relationship-based care approach helped providers in both systems focus on the parent-child relationship, some caregivers noted that providers were not always equipped to meet needs or address issues. Within early intervention, service coordinators were supported with reflective supervision: Supervisors worked closely with service coordinators both to process the experience of working with the family and to develop strategies for the family to move forward. The results suggest that expanded capacity for relationship-based practice in early intervention and behavioral health through training and ongoing support, along with a two-generational approach (i.e., parent and child), can increase engagement in services and treatment across both systems for families experiencing parental depression.

Peer Support and Learning Opportunities. Service providers also benefited from a mechanism referred to as the learning collaborative, which was established to improve their relationship-based approaches through educational support and peer mentoring. Both a group and a process, the learning collaborative allowed providers from the Part C early intervention and behavioral health systems to share experiences and receive regular professional peer contact and support, which helped strengthen individual providers' skill development, knowledge, and comfort level with relationship-based care and allowed for continued interaction and relationship-building with providers from other systems.

Addressing Barriers to Treatment. The initiative also addressed some of the barriers to engagement in behavioral health treatment. The factors of cultural context and stigma were considered during development of the processes for offering depression screening within early intervention and making referrals for behavioral health services and treatment. Cultural framework can affect how individuals communicate about life stressors, their openness to discussing issues, and their willingness to access resources and services. The screening process training for service coordinators, which incorporated discussion and role playing, demonstrated how to affirm the caregiver's feelings, validate their distress, and offer support. The cross-system training sessions and learning collaborative activities emphasized the need to be sensitive to cultural beliefs and concerns when working with families to make referrals and support engagement in services and treatment.

Providing in-home behavioral health services to families in need helped address some of the typical barriers to engaging in treatment, such as lack of transportation, difficulty obtaining child care, the stigma associated with going to a clinic for mental health treatment, and the barrier of depression itself, which can make it difficult to attend traditional outpatient treatment. Community Care and the behavioral health network of providers collaborated to plan an expansion of services that would increase access to and engagement in behavioral health services for this target population. Overall, access to home-based behavioral health services can increase engagement rates and eliminate a significant barrier to accessing behavioral health services.

Individual Outcomes

The assessment of individual outcomes was designed to track caregivers at risk for or experiencing depression and assess their outcomes over time. Outcomes for families involved in the initiative were measured using depression screening measures collected at baseline and at six and 12 months afterward. When a caregiver screened positive for depression, an assessment of parental stress, caregiver health and safety, and child health was administered.

Nearly one-third of caregivers (30 percent) who screened at baseline with the two-question Patient Health Questionnaire (PHQ-2) depression screen also received a six-month follow-up screen. Following the screening protocol, all caregivers who completed the nine-question PHQ-9 at baseline were sought for rescreenings at six and 12 months. Among the 904 caregivers who completed a baseline screen, 16 percent completed a six-month follow-up depression screen (n=149). Overall, few caregivers completed 12-month follow-ups (see Table S.1). There are several possible reasons for the low rates of follow-up in depression screening. Families are discharged from the Part C early intervention system when the child reaches the age of 3 or when the child's functioning has improved to the point where they no longer have a developmental delay. Those discharged were no longer in contact with The Alliance and thus could not be tracked for the follow-up depression screens. Service coordinators also reported that some families declined the follow-up screen because it was stressful to complete during visits with the service coordinator or when there were other service providers in the home.

Nineteen percent of those who took the initial PHQ-2 scored positive. These caregivers were then given the longer PHQ-9 screen. Overall, 9 percent of the caregivers screened positive for depression on the PHQ-9. Studies examining positive screens in low-income mothers report an average rate of 18 percent, with estimates varying across screening tools. Therefore, the initiative population's risk of depression was relatively low by comparison.

Our outcome analysis for those with both baseline and six-month follow-up screens revealed a significant reduction in depressive symptoms both for caregivers who engaged in relationship-based services within the early intervention or behavioral health systems and for those who did not (see Figure S.4). This overall downward trend may reflect a gradual process of adjusting to the stressful situation of identifying a developmental delay for the caregiver's child. The black line in Figure S.4 shows the cut score (10) used to determine depression risk. Both groups were above the cut score at baseline but were, on average, below the cut score at six months.

Assessment of Parental Stress

Those caregivers screening at high risk for depression were asked to complete an assessment that included a parental stress measure as well as caregiver and child health items. A total of 401 caregivers actually completed the assessment, including 290 of the 395 who had screened positive for depression. Results showed that 60 percent of the 290 caregivers who screened positive registered very high levels of parental stress. With respect to different subscales, 79 percent of the sample reached clinical levels of distress on the parental subscale, 37 percent did so on the parent-child dysfunctional interaction subscale, and 45 percent did so on the difficult child subscale.

Our analysis showed that caregivers who completed the assessment at both baseline and follow-up experienced decreased levels of stress. Parental stress scores decreased significantly

Table S.1
Completed Baseline and Follow-Up Depression Screens

Measure	Number Completed at Baseline	Number (%) Completed at Six-Month Follow-Up	Number (%) Completed at 12-Month Follow-Up
PHQ-2	4,185	1252 (30%)	653 (16%)
PHQ-9 (follow-up screen)	904	149 (16%)	88 (10%)
PHQ-9 (positive)	395	94 (24%)	55 (14%)

Figure S.4
Change in PHQ-9 Scores from Baseline to Follow-Up by Engagement

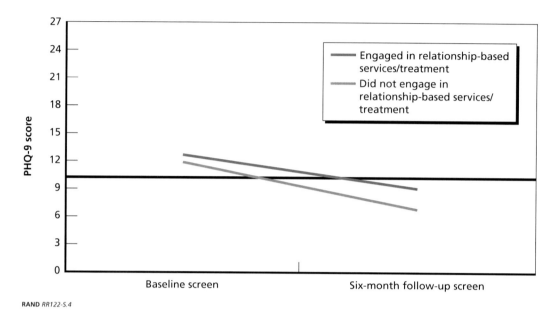

RAND *RR122-S.4*

from baseline to six months and from six months to 12 months both overall and for caregivers who engaged in relationship-based services within the early intervention or behavioral health systems.

Overall, the results of the outcomes analysis suggest that caregivers involved in the initiative experienced better outcomes at six months, regardless of whether they engaged in relationship-based services.

Recommendations

The RAND team built its recommendations off of the *Helping Families Raise Healthy Children* initiative results that have implications for policy and practice in three areas. The recommendations are meant to provide a framework for moving the relevant systems toward a more integrated and coordinated approach to the dual risks of caregiver depression and early childhood developmental delays. Specifically, we offer recommendations to

- improve screening and identification of caregiver depression (Table S.2)
- enhance cross-system referral and coordination (Table S.3)
- increase engagement in services and treatment (Table S.4).

These recommendations are targeted toward decisionmakers and practitioners at the state, county, and provider levels, depending on the jurisdiction. For each area of policy and practice, we present recommendations for the following general groups of stakeholders, with the relevant Pennsylvania entity named in parentheses:

Table S.2
Recommendations to Improve Screening and Identification of Caregiver Depression

Stakeholder	Recommendation
State legislature (Pennsylvania General Assembly)	Mandate universal screening for depression in the Part C early intervention system. Add parental mental health challenges as a qualifying factor for early intervention at-risk tracking services statewide.
State and/or county early intervention agencies (Pennsylvania Department of Public Welfare, Office of Child Development and Early Learning; county early intervention coordination units)	Support referral of infants and toddlers in families with a primary caregiver at risk for depression to early intervention for developmental screening. Add depression as tracking category for early intervention services. Develop protocols for depression screening using a validated screening tool. Provide initial and ongoing training and support on depression screening to service coordinators implementing the screening protocol. Establish performance monitors to assess progress and develop strategies for improving screening rates.
State and/or county behavioral health agencies (Pennsylvania Department of Public Welfare, Office of Mental Health and Substance Abuse Services; county behavioral health administrators)	Support referral of infants and toddlers in families with a primary caregiver experiencing or at risk for depression to early intervention for developmental screening.
Behavioral health provider agencies	Refer infants and toddlers in families with a primary caregiver experiencing or at risk for depression to early intervention for developmental screening. Provide initial and ongoing training and support on caregiver depression, its effect on child development, and the need for developmental screening and assessment for the child.
Providers within the maternal and child health care system	Provide depression screening using a validated tool. Refer infants and toddlers in families with a primary caregiver at risk for depression to early intervention for developmental screening.

- state legislature (Pennsylvania General Assembly)
- state and/or county early intervention agencies (Pennsylvania Department of Public Welfare, Office of Child Development and Early Learning; county early intervention coordination units)
- early intervention provider agencies
- state and/or county behavioral health agencies (Pennsylvania Department of Public Welfare, Office of Mental Health and Substance Abuse Services; county behavioral health administrators)
- behavioral health managed care organizations
- behavioral health provider agencies
- providers within the maternal and child health care system.

Concluding Observation

The *Helping Families Raise Healthy Children* initiative represents a significant step forward in addressing the problem of caregiver depression and childhood developmental risks among families in Allegheny County. Those involved with the initiative will continue efforts to improve care systems within the county and to serve as a catalyst for other communities across the Commonwealth of Pennsylvania.

Table S.3
Recommendations to Enhance Cross-System Referral and Coordination

Stakeholder	Recommendation
State and/or county early intervention agencies (Pennsylvania Department of Public Welfare, Office of Child Development and Early Learning; county early intervention coordination units)	• Promote cross-system collaboration and communication among the early intervention, behavioral health, and maternal and child health care systems. • Develop cross-system referral protocols for families identified as needing behavioral health services and other supports. • Facilitate cross-system collaboration and communication among providers in the early intervention, behavioral health, and maternal and child health care systems. • Provide initial training and ongoing support to service coordinators on cross-system referral protocols. Establish performance monitors to assess progress and develop strategies for improving the cross-system referral process.
Early intervention provider agencies	• Facilitate networking and communication with providers in the behavioral health and maternal and child health care systems.
State and/or county behavioral health agencies (Pennsylvania Department of Public Welfare, Office of Mental Health and Substance Abuse Services; county behavioral health administrators)	• Promote cross-system collaboration and communication among the early intervention, behavioral health, and maternal and child health care systems. • Develop cross-system referral protocols for families identified as needing behavioral health services and other supports. • Facilitate cross-system collaboration and communication among providers in the early intervention, behavioral health, and maternal and child health care systems.
Behavioral health provider agencies	• Facilitate networking and communication with providers in the early intervention and maternal and child health care systems.
Behavioral health managed care organizations	• Support cross-system collaboration and communication among the early intervention, behavioral health, and maternal and child health care systems.

Table S.4
Recommendations to Increase Engagement in Services and Treatment

Stakeholder	Recommendation
State and/or county early intervention agency (Pennsylvania Department of Public Welfare, Office of Child Development and Early Learning; county early intervention coordination units)	• With behavioral health, implement a training curriculum for providers from both systems on the interconnectedness of caregiver depression and early childhood developmental delays, the science of early childhood brain development, the impact of toxic stress, relationship-based care practices, and reflective supervision.
Early intervention provider agencies	• Provide ongoing support and reflective supervision for providers on relationship-based approaches to working with families.
State and/or county behavioral health agencies (Pennsylvania Department of Public Welfare, Office of Mental Health and Substance Abuse Services; county behavioral health administrators	• With early intervention, implement a training curriculum for providers from both systems on the interconnectedness of caregiver depression and early childhood developmental delays, the science of early childhood brain development, the impact of toxic stress, and relationship-based care practices. • Support expansion of in-home behavioral health services for families with caregivers at risk for or experiencing depression and infants/toddlers at risk for developmental delays.
Behavioral health provider agencies	• Expand capacity to provide in-home behavioral health services. • Provide initial and ongoing training and education for providers on relationship-based approaches to working with families.
Behavioral health managed care organizations	• Allow access to in-home behavioral health services for families with caregivers at risk for or experiencing depression and infants/toddlers at risk for developmental delays.

Abbreviations

The Alliance	The Alliance for Infants and Toddlers
The Collaborative	Allegheny County Maternal and Child Health Care Collaborative
Community Care	Community Care Behavioral Health Organization
FAC	Family Advisory Council
IDEA	Individuals with Disabilities Education Act
IFSP	Individualized Family Service Plan
MCO	Managed care organization
PHQ-2	Patient Health Questionnaire (two questions)
PHQ-9	Patient Health Questionnaire (nine questions)
PSI-SF	Parenting Stress Index–Short Form
UPMC	University of Pittsburgh Medical Center
WIC	Women, Infants, and Children

Glossary

Alliance for Infants and Toddlers (The Alliance)	The Allegheny County Department of Human Services contracts with The Alliance to act on its behalf as the single intake, service coordination, and service authorization entity for infants and toddlers (from birth to age three) who may have developmental delays. Their services and responsibilities are specified under Part C of IDEA and PA Early Intervention legislation.
At-risk tracking services	PA Early Intervention legislation provides for infants and toddlers in five specific at-risk categories to be "tracked" until they turn three if they are not currently eligible for an Individualized Family Service Plan. Tracking or monitoring consists of periodic home visits and phone calls to monitor child development and discuss it with the parents. If at any time their screening indicates there are concerns, a full evaluation will be arranged.
Behavioral health system (Allegheny County)	Publicly funded mental health and substance abuse services (behavioral health) are delivered by a large number of agencies under contract with the Allegheny County Department of Human Services and Community Care. Behavioral health services are funded by Medicaid and state/county funds.
Community Care Behavioral Health (Community Care)	In Pennsylvania, counties contract with managed care organizations to manage Medicaid mental health and substance abuse services. Allegheny County contracts with Community Care, a nonprofit behavioral health managed care organization headquartered in Pittsburgh.
Cross-system referral	Referrals for assessment or services across the maternal child health system, the behavioral health system, and the early intervention system.
Early intervention providers	Consultants and agencies/organizations qualified and willing to accept referrals from The Alliance to provide early intervention services as defined in a child's Individualized Family Service Plan.

Early intervention system (Allegheny County)	Pennsylvania designates counties to provide outreach, screening, services coordination, and early intervention services for infants and toddlers in accordance with federal and state laws and regulations. This includes the Individuals with Disabilities Education Act (IDEA) Part C and PA Act 212-1990. The Allegheny County Department of Human Services manages the system and contracts with The Alliance and early intervention providers.
Individualized Family Service Plan (IFSP)	A document developed after a child is determined eligible for early intervention services. Developed by an early intervention service coordinator, early intervention service provider, and the family in a combined effort to meet the developmental needs of children from birth to age three with developmental delay(s).
In-home mobile therapy	Behavioral health services provided by contracted Medicaid behavioral health providers in the consumer's home.
Maternal child health system (Allegheny County)	A wide range of providers in Allegheny County addressing the health and quality of life of mothers and their infants/children. This includes the maternity programs of the Medicaid physical health managed care organizations, pediatricians, the Allegheny County Health Department and numerous maternal and child health care agencies. Services are funded by the Title V Mother and Child Health Coalition, Healthy Start, Medicaid, human services funding, and state funds from the Pennsylvania Departments of Public Welfare and Health.
Mental health specialist	Professionals with advanced degrees and training in promoting infant-caregiver relationships in order to provide optimal social-emotional development. These grant-funded employees at The Alliance provided ongoing support and consultation to service coordinators on the screening and referral processes, provided a direct contact and outreach to behavioral health providers, and assisted in the design and implementation of most aspects of the initiative.
Part C	Part C is the section of the Federal Individuals with Disabilities Education Act (IDEA) that provides for a federal grant program to states that assists states in operating a comprehensive statewide program for early intervention services for children from birth to age three with disabilities. The program was created to enhance the development of infants and toddlers and the capacity of families to meet their child's needs. The Program for Infants and Toddlers with Disabilities (Part C) contains many requirements states have to meet, including the minimum components of their system.
Reflective supervision	Supervision that encourages mutual sharing, reflecting, and planning between the supervisor and the service provider.

Relationship-based care	Therapies/services that help parents interpret and respond to their infants' cues, express their own emotions, and prevent or repair damage to the parent-child relationship. This approach is grounded in attachment models with emphasis on parallel processes such that what happens in one set of relationships will be mirrored in other relationships (i.e., the provider's way of being with and relating to the caregiver will eventually be replicated in the way the caregiver relates to the child).
Relationship-based service coordination	A way for service coordinators within early intervention to engage with families and recognize the relationship as a driving force for change within the family unit. This approach focuses on supporting the relationship of caregiver and child to enhance delivery and long-term outcomes of early intervention services.
Service coordinator	Alliance employees who work with families of children with developmental delays to set goals, monitor the child's development and progress, monitor services the child is receiving, provide parent support and education, and assist in the transition to appropriate services at age three.
Team-delivered, in-home behavioral health services	A comprehensive set of services provided by a team composed of a mental health professional and a mental health worker that includes referrals and linkages to other services as needed for Medicaid-eligible families; also known in Allegheny County as Family Focused Solution Based services.

CHAPTER ONE

Introduction

Starting in August 2009, a group of partners in the Pittsburgh area involved with the behavioral health and Part C early intervention systems undertook an effort to improve care for families at risk for the dual challenges of caregiver depression and early childhood developmental delays. This effort—called *Helping Families Raise Healthy Children*—was conducted under the auspices of the Allegheny County Maternal and Child Health Care Collaborative, a broad-based community coalition that has been operating since January 2002. This report describes the initiative, including the impetus behind it and its planning and implementation processes, and presents the results and lessons learned from a comprehensive evaluation of the program's implementation. It concludes with recommendations for practice and policy change designed to expand and sustain the initiative's achievements.

Background on the Allegheny County Maternal and Child Health Care Collaborative

Allegheny County, which includes the city of Pittsburgh, is a community rich in health care resources. Nevertheless, the region has its shortcomings: high rates of women receiving no prenatal care in the first trimester (112 per 1,000 pregnancies); high rates of infants born at low birth weight (80 births per 1,000); high infant mortality rates (7.6 per 1,000 live births); particularly among African-American infants (15.1 per 1,000 live births); and mothers and young children with poor health outcomes in a number of key areas (Commonwealth of Pennsylvania, 2012). Nationally, the infant mortality rate was 6.15 in 2010 (National Center for Health Statistics, 2012). Faced with this continuing evidence of poor health outcomes and racial disparities, as well as the documented negative lifelong consequences and high costs associated with low birth weight and lack of prenatal care (Institute of Medicine, 2007), stakeholders in Allegheny County recognized the deficiencies and need for change in the local system of maternal and child health care.

In recognition of the important role that community coalitions can play in the health system reform process (Institute of Medicine, 2001; Adams, Greiner, and Corrigan, 2004; Gostin, Boufford, and Martinez, 2004), The Heinz Endowments, a large Pittsburgh foundation, commissioned the RAND–University of Pittsburgh Health Institute in January 2002 to organize the Allegheny County Maternal and Child Health Care Collaborative. In partnership with the Allegheny County Department of Health and the Allegheny County Department of Human Services, a project team led by RAND brought together all key systems partners in a collaborative effort to build a model system of care for mothers and young children in the region. Drawing on the basic tenets of systems change put forth by the Institute of Medicine (2001, 2006) and adapted in related evidence-based efforts to improve systems performance (Wagner, 1998; Wagner et al., 2001), the Collaborative began an effort to transform systems for mothers and young children in Allegheny County.

The Collaborative's Prior Work

Phase I: Planning Process, 2002–2004

In the two years following establishment of the Collaborative, all systems partners—including consumers and families, physical health practices and providers, health plans, and local and state purchasers and policymakers—engaged in a systematic planning process designed to transform the Collaborative's vision of an ideal maternal and child health care system into a focused strategy and action plan. Attention was paid to both the practices and policies of systems change, leading to a plan with several key goals:

- Develop an established medical or social service home for each family in the community.
- Promote a family-centered, culturally competent approach to care in which providers address the needs, and draw on the strengths, of the entire family being served.
- Provide integrated/holistic services, with service providers working closely together, addressing all aspects of a family's health and social needs that affect the child at risk for developmental delays.
- Develop a high-quality maternal and child health care workforce, well trained in the principles of family-centered care, cultural competence, and integrated/holistic care.
- Inform families about available programs and resources, educate them about health behaviors, and empower them to demand high-quality maternal and child health care.
- Promote effective leadership at the state and county levels with clear lines of authority and accountability for performance.

The Collaborative identified four priority areas for improvement: prenatal care, family behavioral health, nutrition, and chronic illness and special health care needs. The Collaborative also identified two domains of best practice, family engagement and care coordination/service integration, to be adapted and implemented in the community.

Our research explored the barriers to adoption of these best practices in relation to the targeted areas for improvement, and ways to overcome them. The results of these efforts are documented in a previous RAND monograph titled *Improving Maternal and Child Health Care: A Blueprint for Community Action in the Pittsburgh Region* (Pincus et al., 2005).

Phase II: Pilot Testing, 2004–2006

Using the blueprint as a guide, the Collaborative designed a one-year pilot study to test whether several small-scale versions of its proposed evidence-based practice approach to systems improvement would be realistic and workable in local community settings. In addition, the Collaborative determined the specific types of policy and health systems changes that would be required to enhance and sustain these efforts. The pilot, carried out between October 2004 and September 2005, involved three community-based improvement teams focused on three of the Collaborative's priority areas for improvement: prenatal care, maternal depression, and childhood obesity.

The results of these efforts are documented in a 2006 RAND report produced by the Collaborative entitled *Building a Model Maternal and Child Health Care System in the Pittsburgh Region: A Community-Based Quality Improvement Initiative* (Allegheny County Maternal and Child Health Care Collaborative, 2006). Results varied across measures and teams, but the gap between local physical and behavioral health care systems emerged as a sentinel issue underlying many of the ongoing maternal and child health care challenges. This finding highlighted the need for continued efforts to coordinate and integrate care, particularly in the context of high-priority areas that crosscut both systems, such as maternal depression.

Phase III: Maternal Depression Initiative, 2007–2010

Based on the results of the pilot study, the third phase of the Collaborative's work focused on maternal depression. The Allegheny County Maternal Depression Initiative aimed to improve the capacity of the local physical health and behavioral health systems for identifying women at high risk for maternal depression, enhancing their access to available resources and services, and engaging them in behavioral health treatment as needed. With support and leadership from the University of Pittsburgh Medical Center (UPMC) Health Plan and the Allegheny County Department of Human Services, Office of Behavioral Health, the initiative worked with physical health providers to screen pregnant and postpartum women for risk of depression, refer women who screened positive to physical health care managers from their managed care organization, and support their engagement in behavioral health treatment.

The results of these efforts are documented in a 2010 RAND report entitled *Building Bridges: Lessons from a Pittsburgh Partnership to Strengthen Systems of Care for Maternal Depression* (Keyser et al., 2010). While difficult to disentangle specific cause-and-effect relationships among the initiative strategies and the outcomes that were achieved, the results indicate that the Collaborative was successful in improving key organizational and clinical processes related to screening, referral, and engagement in treatment for pregnant and postpartum women, particularly as compared with rates of maternal depression screening, referral, and engagement in treatment found in the literature. In other areas, the Collaborative confronted challenges. For example, it was difficult to ensure consistent and timely communication among those with shared responsibility for high-risk women. Further, there was a considerable lag between a woman's identification and referral and her ultimate engagement in behavioral health treatment, representing a target for continued quality improvement over time. The findings from this initiative highlighted the need for continued efforts to improve coordination and collaboration of care for women at high risk for depression, particularly around screening, referral, and engagement in behavioral health treatment.

The Broad Context for the Collaborative's Focus on Depression

Each year, more than 2,500 infants and toddlers in Allegheny County are referred for Part C early intervention services due to concerns about communication, cognitive, social/emotional, or developmental issues that can harm their future learning, behavior, and health (Pennsylvania State Interagency Coordinating Council, 2010–2011). Up to 60 percent of these very young children are estimated to have mothers at increased risk for depression due to adverse life circumstances, including poverty, lack of social supports, and stress linked to hardship (Administration for Children and Families, 2006; Kahn et al., 1999; Siefert et al., 2000). Research shows that healthy early childhood development is directly linked to the quality of the parent-child relationship (Davies, Winter, and Cicchetti, 2006; Sroufe et al., 2005), and that maternal depression poses a serious risk to this relationship and, in turn, healthy child development (Cummings et al., 2008; Elgar et al., 2007; Goodman and Gotlib, 1999; Lim, Wood, and Miller, 2008). Conversely, a child's developmental delays can increase maternal stress, heightening risk for depression (Davis et al., 2003; Singer et al., 1999; Singer, 2006). Screening, referral, and engagement in services and treatment for maternal depression early in a child's development may offset this negative cycle and improve outcomes for both children and their caregivers. Yet, as the 2009 Institute of Medicine's Consensus Report emphasized, "the delivery of adequate screening and successful detection and treatment of a depressive illness and prevention of its effects on parenting and the health of children is a formidable challenge to modern health care systems" (National Research Council and Institute of Medicine, 2009).

Prevalence and Symptoms of Maternal Depression

Depression affects more than 18 million Americans each year, and is much more likely to affect women. Researchers estimate that, in any given year, depressive illnesses affect 12 percent of women and nearly 7 percent of men (Narrow, 1998). For most individuals, depression is characterized by cycles of relapse and remittance over a lifetime. On average, adults who have one episode of major depression will have at least five episodes across their lifetime (Pepper and Maack, 2009). About 20 percent of those who recover from an episode (remission of symptoms for at least eight weeks) will have a recurrence within one year; the rate of recurrence increases with subsequent episodes (Pepper and Maack, 2009). Common symptoms of depression include prolonged periods of depressed or irritable mood, fatigue, loss of interest in activities, changes in sleep or appetite, feelings of guilt or worthlessness, or thoughts of harming oneself or someone else.

Women in their reproductive period (ages 15 to 45) are twice as likely to suffer from depression as men in the same age group (Kessler et al., 1994; Gaynes et al., 2005). Prevalence of depression ranges from 8.5 to 11 percent during pregnancy and from 6.5 to 12.9 percent during the first year postpartum (Gaynes et al., 2005). Recent studies investigating the stability and change of depressive symptoms in low-income mothers found that most mothers demonstrate stable levels of depression (both low symptoms and clinical levels of symptoms) during the first couple of years after childbirth, suggesting the importance of screening at-risk women early during pregnancy and offering services to connect women to needed treatment (Beeghly et al., 2002; Beeghly et al., 2003; Mora et al., 2009; Ramos-Marcuse et al., 2010).

Prevalence and Risk Factors of Maternal Depression for Low-Income Populations

Among low-income and other underserved populations (e.g., minority women), the estimated prevalence rates for maternal depression are much higher, typically ranging from 25 to 35 percent (Lanzi et al., 1999; Miranda and Green, 1999; Onunaku, 2005; Siefert et al., 2000), which is markedly higher than depression rates of the general population, as previously discussed. Findings from the Early Childhood Longitudinal Study found that maternal depression disproportionately affects children in low-income families. Specifically, 25 percent of mothers with family incomes less than or equal to 100 percent of the poverty level were moderately or severely depressed (Center on the Developing Child at Harvard University, 2009). This is in contrast to

19 percent and 11 percent of mothers whose family income was between 100 and 200 percent of the poverty level or more than 200 percent above it, respectively. According to analysis of data from the Pregnancy Risk Assessment Monitoring System 3 for 2004–2005, the average prevalence of self-reported postpartum depressive symptoms among women who received Medicaid benefits for their delivery was 21 percent (Centers for Disease Control and Prevention, 2008).

These high rates of prevalence among low-income women are often linked to life circumstances, which encompass many of the main risk factors for maternal depression. These risk factors include, but are not limited to, individual or family history of depression (Robertson et al., 2004), history of alcohol dependence or other substance use (Ross and Dennis, 2009), extreme social stressors and poor marital relationships (Ramchandani and Psychogiou, 2009), lack of social support or absence of a community network (Ingram and Taylor, 2007; Robertson et al., 2004), childhood trauma and past or current experiences of intimate-partner violence (Knitzer, Theberge, and Johnson, 2008), and unplanned or unwanted pregnancy (O'Hara and Swain, 1996).

Prevention and Intervention Effects for Women At Risk for Depression

Generally, early prevention and intervention efforts for depression are effective at reducing risk for depression among mothers (Barlow and Coren, 2004; Cooper et al., 2003; Miller et al., 2008; Murray et al., 2003; Sockol, Epperson, and Barber, 2011; Van der Waerden, Hoefnagels, and Hosman, 2011), as well as for low-income or other high-risk mothers (Beeber et al., 2004; Dennis et al., 2009; Laperriere et al., 2005; Lara et al., 2003; Lipman and Boyle, 2005; Peden, 2005; Wiggins et al., 2005). Although types of interventions vary (e.g., nurse-delivered in-home psychotherapy, group cognitive-behavioral therapy, community-based social support and education groups), evaluations of interventions for low-income women at risk for depression consistently find treatment effects up to one year post-intervention. However, such effects are rarely maintained beyond this first year (e.g., Peden, 2005; Wiggins et al., 2005). These findings suggest that the cumulative effect of stressors in the home environment may prove difficult to overcome and can interfere with sustaining practices learned while receiving treatment (Van der Waerden, Hoefnagels, and Hosman, 2011).

Link Between Maternal Depression and Early Childhood Development

Untreated maternal depression has potentially serious consequences for a woman's overall well-being, her functioning as a mother, the family's functioning, and her child's development (Onunaku, 2005; Field, 2000). It poses a serious risk for healthy child development by compromising the quality of the parent-child relationship during critical years of development (Cummings et al., 2008; Elgar et al., 2007; Goodman and Gotlib, 1999; Lim, Wood, and Miller, 2008; Lovejoy et al., 2000). Healthy brain development during early childhood requires a "serve and return" pattern of interactions between caregivers and their infants (Center on the Developing Child at Harvard University, 2009; Tronick, 2007). These interactions help develop key connections in the child's brain that aids in the healthy formation of the stress response systems, language formation, and other cognitive skills. However, depression may interfere with a caregiver's ability to engage in these interactions (Center on the Developing Child at Harvard University, 2009; Tronick, 2007). Specifically, depressed caregivers often display one of two problematic patterns of parenting—(1) hostile and/or intrusive, or (2) disengaged or withdrawn—that disrupt the "serve and return" interaction essential for healthy brain development (Center on the Developing Child at Harvard University, 2009). Depressed mothers also generally show less attentiveness and responsiveness to their children's needs and are less likely to use preventive services (Diego, Field, and Hernandez-Reif, 2005). Moreover, a child's developmental delays can increase maternal stress, ultimately increasing risk for depression and perpetuating a cycle that affects both mother and child (Davis et al., 2003; Singer, 2006; Singer et al., 1999).

Exposure to maternal depression and the associated "toxic stress" has grave consequences for healthy child development. Perinatal depression, in particular, affects children prenatally and after birth (Bonari et al., 2004). Depressed women are more likely to give birth prematurely, and their infants are at greater risk of being small for gestational age (U.S. Department of Health and Human Services, Office of Women's Health, 2009). After birth, a mother's ability to bond with her child might also be compromised by depression, placing infants at risk for delayed social and emotional development (Diego, Field, and Hernandez-Reif, 2005; Paulson, Dauber, and Leiferman, 2006; Murray and Cooper, 1997). Children of depressed mothers experience more social and emotional problems than children whose mothers are not depressed (Moore, Cohn, and Campbell, 2001; Whitaker, Orzol, and Kahn, 2006). Delays or impairments in cognitive and linguistic development and social interactions also emerge (Grace, Evindar, and Stewart, 2003; Downey and Coyne, 1990). Children of mothers with continued depression are more likely to develop long-term behavioral problems and are at greater risk of developing psychopathology, including affective (mainly depression), anxiety, and conduct disorders, later in life (Beck, 1999; Weissman et al., 2006).

As such, the dual challenges of maternal depression and child developmental delay pose unique threats to both the mother and child. Children with developmental delays may require greater levels of responsiveness and engagement from mothers to meet the daily challenges associated with physical health problems, cognitive delays, and behavioral problems. Depression may hinder a mother's ability to provide these additional supports to her children. Additionally, the stress of managing the added needs of a child with a developmental delay, as well as concern about long-term outcomes, may exacerbate or prolong depression in mothers. Early childhood developmental delays combined with ongoing exposure to maternal depression can result in negative long-term outcomes, such as poor physical health, poor academic performance, depression and other psychological disorders, delinquent behavior, and conduct problems (Goodman and Gotlib, 1999). Intensive intervention efforts that focused specifically on mother-child interactions have shown improved developmental outcomes among children of depressed mothers (Cicchetti, Rogosch, and Toth, 2000), as well as improved interactions between mother and child (Clark, Tluczek, and Wenzel, 2003; Cicchetti, Rogosch, and Toth, 2000). Initiating screening, referral for treatment, and engagement in treatment for maternal depression early in a child's life may offset this negative cycle and improve outcomes for both mothers and their children (Cicchetti, Rogosch, and Toth, 2000; Clark, Tluczek, and Wenzel, 2003). Moreover, using a two-generation approach (i.e., parent and child) with mothers at risk for or experiencing depression may help them cope with the parenting challenges of having a child with developmental delays, while offering enhanced support for the child.

System Challenges to Addressing Maternal Depression

Although the dual challenges of maternal depression and children's developmental delays often co-occur (Sohr-Preston and Scaramella, 2006), the relevant care systems in the United

States typically identify and treat them separately. These systems have evolved in a manner that fosters specialization and fragmentation in treatment and interventions. Lillas and Turnbull point out that "often families end up enlisting the help of a variety of practitioners in a serial fashion, presenting their child's same problems yet hearing interpretations through a different professional lens inadvertently culminating in a confusing, distressing and disheartening scenario" (2009, p. 7). This fragmentation can result in families having multiple comprehensive treatment plans, unrelated interventions, repeating their story countless times to different providers, and interacting with a variety of therapists in a variety of settings. Early intervention services traditionally focus on addressing the specific developmental delays experienced by children and may not consider the emotional impact on parents or the adult's need for support and services. Conversely, behavioral health providers, physical health providers, and community agencies that serve adults with depression often do not consider the impact of parental depression on young children in the family or focus on the adult's role as a parent. Furthermore, settings focused on children (e.g., pediatric offices or early intervention programs) tend to lack established systematic practices for identifying maternal depression; this, along with the lack of coordinated referral between pediatric and adult systems, impedes the ability of providers to connect depressed mothers with appropriate services. As a result, many mothers do not receive the supports and services they need to manage both their depression and their children's developmental needs, which may place the health and well-being of the entire family at risk.

Maternal Depression Screening
Although systematic screening is now widely recognized as a necessary prerequisite for the early identification of maternal depression, few pediatric primary care physicians report using a validated tool at specified intervals to screen for maternal depression (Heneghan, Morton, and DeLeone, 2007; Olson et al., 2002; LaRocco-Cockburn et al., 2003; Seehusen et al., 2005). Overall, maternal depression screening rates average around 38 percent (e.g., Armstrong and Small, 2007; Garcia, LaCaze, and Ratanasen, 2011; LaRocco-Cockburn et al., 2003; Seehusen et al., 2005; Segre et al., 2011). However, estimates vary widely depending on health care setting, with rates of 8 percent for pediatricians (Heneghan, Morton, and DeLeone, 2007; Olson et al., 2002), 24 percent for obstetricians (La-Rocco-Cockburn et al., 2003), and 31 percent for family medicine physicians (Seehusen et al., 2005). Recent results from chart reviews of Health Choice members conducted by Pennsylvania's Office of Medical Assistance Programs indicate rates of prenatal depression screening ranged from 51 percent in 2008 to 65 percent in 2009, and postpartum depression screening ranged from 34 percent in 2008 to 51 percent in 2009 (OMAP, 2008–2009). However, because the rates do not distinguish physicians who use validated screening tools from those who rely on non-standardized screening methods, percentages are likely inflated.

When providers use a validated tool to screen for maternal depression, estimates of positive screens range from 6 to 57 percent, with an average rate of 30 percent for low-income populations (e.g., Beeber et al., 2010; Bethell, Peck, and Schor, 2001; Birndorf et al., 2001; Carter et al., 2005; Goodman and Tyer-Viola, 2010; Marcus et al., 2003; Miller, Shade, and Vasireddy, 2009; Olson et al., 2005; Shim et al., 2011; Smith et al., 2004). However, rates vary depending on the setting (primary care vs. early intervention), the patient population (low-income, predominantly minority patients) and screening tools (e.g., the nine-question Patient Health Questionnaire [PHQ-9], Beck Depression Inventory, Center for Epidemiologic Studies

Depression Scale). OMAP (2008, 2009) reports of positive screens during prenatal or post-partum depression screening echoed peer-reviewed reports and ranged from 17 to 30 percent.

Despite recent recommendations to screen for maternal depression in primary care settings, more than 75 percent of pediatric primary care physicians still rely on behavior, appearance, and complaints to recognize depression (Heneghan, Morton, and DeLeone, 2007; Olson et al., 2002). Additionally, when providers do screen for depression, they often use their own questions about mood or mental health to recognize depression rather than validated screening tools (LaRocco-Cockburn et al., 2003). Such practices raise concerns given findings indicating poor accuracy among pediatric providers in recognizing depression without the use of a validated screening tool (Heneghan et al., 2000). For instance, when screening in the health care setting is based on clinical observation alone, 50 percent of women suffering from depression are missed (Wilen and Mounts, 2006). These barriers, along with other provider-level barriers (e.g., lack of training in identifying signs of depression in diverse populations), ultimately result in poor identification of women who are depressed.

Actions Taken Following Positive Screens

Depression screening alone has yet to be linked directly to improvement in depression (Gaynes et al., 2005). To be effective, screening must be followed by a formal diagnostic assessment, a method to guide referral or treatment decisions, and quality monitoring to track and remedy unexpected developments (Miller, Shade, and Vasireddy, 2009). Survey estimates of referral rates following a positive depression screen at well-child visits average approximately 50 percent (e.g., Chaudron et al., 2004; Sheeder, Kabir, and Stafford, 2009; Yonkers et al., 2009), ranging from 20 percent to upward of 73 percent (Goodman and Tyer-Viola, 2010; OMAP, 2008). However, rates vary considerably by setting and available follow-up services (e.g., Chaudron et al., 2004; Goodman and Tyer-Viola, 2010; Olson et al., 2005; Olson et al., 2006). Reports of referrals in primary care health settings tend to represent the lower range of referral rates (e.g., Goodman and Tyer-Viola, 2010; Olson et al., 2005), whereas referrals from early intervention settings have been higher, at around 50 percent (Chaudron et al., 2004). For providers, the lack of a triage process to refer and treat individuals who screen positive for depression is a major barrier to connecting caregivers with services in the mental health system (Boyd et al., 2011; Children's Defense Fund of Minnesota, 2011). Further, a lack of established communication channels between the adult behavioral health care system and the pediatric health care system makes coordination across systems difficult (Abrams, Dornig, and Curran, 2009; Boyd et al., 2011; Children's Defense Fund of Minnesota, 2011).

Engagement in Behavioral Health Treatment

Treatments for maternal depression reach only a small subset of depressed women. This is especially true for racial and ethnic minorities, who have less access to mental health services and are less likely to receive high-quality mental health care (Agency for Healthcare Research and Quality, 2004; Skaer et al., 2000; Wang, Berglund, and Kessler, 2000; Young et al., 2001; Vesga-López et al., 2008). Based on the few studies or interventions of screening and referral systems that report engagement rates for low-income women, the average engagement rate was approximately 37 percent (Miranda et al., 2003; Sit et al., 2009; Smith et al., 2009; Wiggins et al., 2005). Estimates of engagement in at least one session following referral for services ranged from approximately 16 percent up to 94 percent (Miranda et al., 2003; Sit et al., 2009; Wiggins et al., 2005), with rates varying considerably by types of follow-up services.

In addition to challenges to access, caregivers' negative beliefs about mental illness and treatment, as well as personal constraints (e.g., childcare, transportation), prove to be major barriers to treatment (Abrams, Dornig, and Curran, 2009; Sit and Wisner, 2009), and may be particularly salient for low-income minority women. Among those who do engage in treatment, discontinuities in care during pregnancy and postpartum can complicate the recovery process (Bennett et al., 2010). These discontinuities might be exacerbated by a lack of coordination between care providers (American Congress of Obstetricians and Gynecologists, 2006), as well as the fact that many health care providers are uncomfortable treating depression without input from mental health care providers (LaRocco-Cockburn et al., 2003; Hill et al., 2001; Dietrich et al., 2003).

Sustaining engagement in treatment long enough to observe positive change in outcomes is another challenge, as is defining what constitutes an "adequate dose" of treatment for maternal depression. In their recent review of the availability of treatment for maternal depression, Witt and colleagues (2009) defined adequate dose as receipt of at least eight 30-minute outpatient or office-based psychotherapy visits or at least four antidepressant prescriptions. Other studies have shown that the percentage of patients who report improvements in their symptoms of depression doubles between zero and three doses (Howard et al., 1986). When looking at studies on engagement for low-income women who received multiple sessions of treatment (i.e., engagement in more than one session), rates of engagement were low, ranging from 6 percent of mothers from publically funded obstetric clinics who received services from a community mental health care clinicians to 17 percent of mothers screened initially at Women, Infants and Children (WIC) programs who received services from community mental health care clinicians (Smith et al., 2009; Miranda et al., 2003). These low rates of engagement in multiple sessions may suggest that caregivers find it difficult to attend multiple sessions while juggling multiple stressors and demands at home. For these reasons, a formal system that provides routine depression screening with a validated tool, appropriate referrals when needed, and support to address the barriers to treatment is needed.

The Need for a Cross-System Response to Maternal Depression in Allegheny County

At the outset of the initiative, the local systems in Allegheny County were set up to serve children at risk for developmental delays and parents at risk for or experiencing depression as if the conditions and target populations were independent of each other (Figure 1.1). Each year approximately 2,500 children in Allegheny County are referred to the Part C early intervention system, with most of them either identified as having or determined to be at risk for developmental delays (Pennsylvania State Interagency Coordinating Council, 2010–2011). At the same time, an estimated 6,000 infants are born to women enrolled in Medicaid in Allegheny County each year, of which approximately 1,800 have a primary caregiver with depression. Given the documented interconnectedness of parental depression and early childhood developmental delays, as well as the prevalence of these outcomes in the community, it was expected that significant numbers of the caregivers at risk for or experiencing depression would have children either experiencing or at risk for developmental delays, and that many of the children referred for developmental delays would have parents experiencing or at increased risk for depression.

Figure 1.1
Existing Public Systems for Early Childhood Developmental Delays and Caregiver Depression

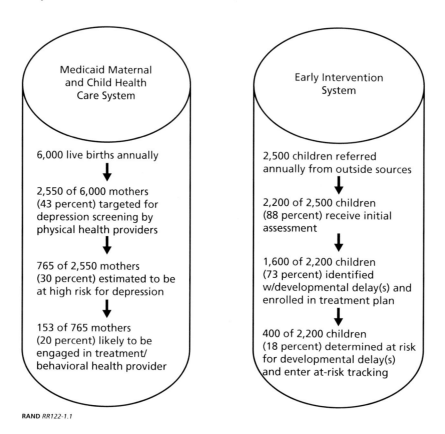

RAND *RR122-1.1*

The federal Individuals with Disabilities Education Improvement Act (IDEA) of 2004 Program for Infants and Toddlers with Disabilities (Part C) provides a federal grant program that assists states in operating comprehensive programs for early intervention services for children up to three years of age with disabilities. The program was created to enhance the development of infants and toddlers and the capacity of families to meet their child's needs. Part C contains many requirements states have to meet, including specifying the minimum components of their system. Part C supports many opportunities for local collaboration in caring for very young children, and Pennsylvania's relatively progressive requirements for early intervention (25 percent delay or clinical opinion) have enabled interventions for a significant 73 percent of children who are assessed for developmental delays. Beyond that, the development of infants/toddlers not currently eligible for intervention services can be monitored over time if certain risk factors are present. However, the Part C legislation does not provide for parental depression screening within the early intervention system, nor does it recognize parental depression as an eligible risk factor for tracking services for early childhood development. Moreover, there were no established practices for cross-referrals of parents and children from early intervention to either Medicaid mental health services or non-public mental health services within the maternal and child health care system. As a result, hundreds of opportunities to identify at-risk parents and infants/toddlers and engage them in appropriate care across the different systems were being missed.

The *Helping Families Raise Healthy Children* Initiative

Aims and Focus of the Initiative

Helping Families Raise Healthy Children represents the Collaborative's next step in achieving its vision of a model maternal and child health care system. The initiative focuses on identifying at-risk families, integrating and coordinating services across systems, and building system capacity while embodying the Collaborative's strategic vision for system improvement and occupying the domains of best practice outlined in the Phase 1 planning process. Further, consistent with the Institute of Medicine's recommendations, *Helping Families Raise Healthy Children* is a two-generation (i.e., parents and their children), cross-systems quality improvement initiative that employs a relationship-based approach to service delivery. For early intervention and behavioral health providers, relationship-based services help parents interpret and respond to their infants' cues, express their own emotions, and prevent or repair damage to the parent-child relationship. For service coordinators at The Alliance, relationship-based service coordination engages families and supports the relationship of caregiver and child to enhance delivery and long-term outcomes of early intervention services. Overall, the initiative was designed to ensure that both caregivers and infants are well served by integrating the local Part C early intervention system for infants and toddlers with the infrastructure that supports adult behavioral health care. This approach addresses early childhood development and maternal depression in the context of the parent-child relationship. *Helping Families Raise Healthy Children* has three main objectives:

- improve identification of families with primary caregivers at risk for or experiencing depression and infants/toddlers at risk for or experiencing developmental delays
- enhance access to support and services for these families through referrals for assessment or services in the Medicaid maternal and child health, behavioral health, and early intervention systems
- offer and support engagement in relationship-based services that address the needs of both caregivers and young children in the context of the parent-child relationship.

The initiative's implementation strategy was designed to achieve sustainable improvements in processes (e.g., screening, referral, and engagement) and outcomes (e.g., caregiver depression) by providing better understanding and response to families' needs and preferences; establishing a cross-system collaborative network; improving providers' capacity to deliver relationship-based care; and establishing cross-system practices for these efforts. To this end, three components of service delivery were targeted for improvement at the systems level:

1. screening and identification of at-risk families through three pathways within and between the Part C early intervention system and the maternal and child health care system
2. referrals for those identified as being at risk
3. engagement in relationship-based services in both the Part C early intervention and behavioral health systems.

Roles and Responsibilities of Key Stakeholder Groups

To achieve the initiative's three aims, the Collaborative convened seven stakeholder groups to work together. These groups and their roles and responsibilities in relation to the aims of the initiative are as follows:

- Families at dual risk for depression and early childhood developmental delays were the target population of the initiative. During the planning and implementation phases, this group provided advice on the initiative implementation protocols, strategies, and materials through a Family Advisory Council (FAC).
- Community Care Behavioral Health Organization (Community Care), the Medicaid behavioral health managed care organization (MCO), provided care management and ensures access to available resources and services for identified families, to increase the likelihood that they would effectively engage in behavioral health treatment as needed and appropriate. Community Care provided the organizational and project leadership and facilitated the involvement of the behavioral health network of providers.
- The Alliance for Infants and Toddlers (The Alliance) is the central intake and service coordination unit for families of children (birth to three years of age). It screened and identified families at high risk for depression and took steps to link them to available supports, services, and treatments as needed and appropriate. The Alliance also educated and supported all service coordinators in a relationship-based approach to service coordination.
- Early intervention service provider organizations (birth to three years of age) provided in-home, relationship-based services for children with developmental delays.
- Behavioral health provider organizations offered a range of well-established treatments that meet the needs and preferences of the referred families with very young children. Community Care developed a network of behavioral health providers able to offer home-based mental health treatment services for families receiving Medicaid.
- Maternal and child health care providers and organizations in the community identified families at high risk for depression and referred them to The Alliance for screening and developmental assessment.
- State and local purchasers and policymakers supported practice and policy changes to enhance the ability of systems partners to carry out their agreed-upon roles.

Other organizations in the community offered support (e.g., funding, data collection and analysis, access to requisite resources and services outside the maternal and child health care system) to ensure successful and sustainable systems change.

Figure 1.2 provides a high-level overview of the relationships among these groups with respect to identifying families at risk for caregiver depression (aim 1), enhancing their access to available resources and services (aim 2), and supporting their engagement in relationship-based services in the Part C early intervention and behavioral systems as needed and appropriate (aim 3).

Through the active engagement and commitment of these key stakeholders, this community-based collaborative aimed to create a new cadre of service professionals who can bridge the gap between the adult mental health and Part C early intervention systems. The goal was to build a sustainable cross-systems infrastructure that improved local capacity to identify and engage families with caregivers at risk for or experiencing depression and children at risk for

Figure 1.2.
Key Stakeholder Groups for the *Helping Families Raise Healthy Children* Initiative

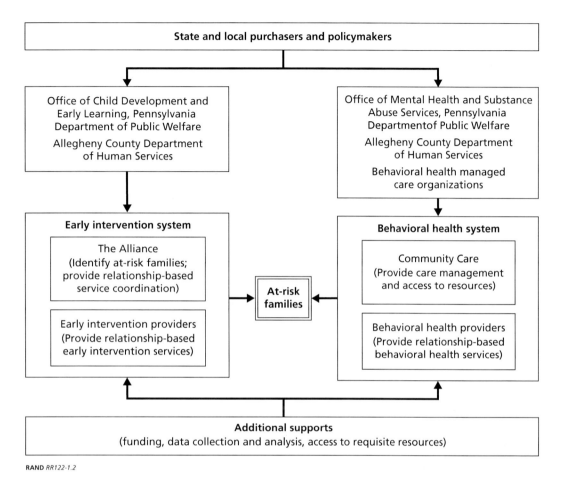

developmental delays, and to change practice and policy so that more parents are empowered to provide their children with opportunities to reach their fullest potential and, in so doing, enhance their own prospects for improved health and well-being.

Strategies for Implementation

Together with the Collaborative, the three organizing partners for the initiative (Community Care, The Alliance, and RAND) developed protocols and procedures for implementing the initiative's components of screening and identification, referral, and engagement in relationship-based services. The project team also designed and implemented a comprehensive set of strategies to support the partners in fulfilling their roles and responsibilities. These strategies included cross-system provider education and training, a learning collaborative group and process for providers in both the Part C early intervention system and the behavioral health system, community outreach, and an FAC. Details on the initiative implementation protocol and strategies are provided in Chapter Two.

Initiative Timeline

The *Helping Families Raise Healthy Children* initiative began on August 1, 2009, and officially ended data collection on May 31, 2012. The initiative's work was conducted in four phases:

Start-up phase (August 2009–January 2010). Protocols and procedures for screening and referrals were developed. Service coordinators and supervisors at The Alliance were trained on the depression screening and referral protocols. Community Care worked with behavioral health providers to develop capacity for home-based mobile mental health treatment services and expanded existing relationship-based services for the initiative's target population.

Phase 1 implementation (February 2010–January 2011). Screening and referral components were implemented. Workshops were held for early intervention and behavioral health providers on relationship-based services and approaches. For the evaluation, RAND collected process data on the screening, referral, and engagement in treatment components; system impact data on the cross-systems trainings; and individual outcome data from caregivers completing the screening and assessment process. RAND also conducted interim data analyses to inform ongoing implementation.

Phase 2 implementation (February 2011–May 2012). Implementation of the screening and referral components continued, as did additional workshops on relationship-based approaches. This phase incorporated the relationship-based approaches within the Part C early intervention and behavioral health systems for those identified as at risk for or experiencing depression. RAND continued to collect process, system impact, and individual outcome data and to provide interim analyses to inform ongoing quality improvement.

Reporting and dissemination (June 2012–June 2013). RAND analyzed the results of the data collection, and the results were used to develop recommendations for sustaining practice and policy improvements. The results were also disseminated to community stakeholders via this report, national and local conferences, and a planned public policy forum. The project team also worked on integrating the implementation components to sustainable practices across the involved systems and developed an implementation toolkit for other communities interested in depression screening, referral, and treatment across systems (Schultz et al., 2012).

Organization of This Report

This report presents the data gathered for the initiative's multifaceted evaluation. Chapter Two describes the methods for achieving the three aims of the *Helping Families Raise Healthy Children* initiative. Chapter Three assesses implementation of the screening, referral, and engagement-in-services components of the initiative and presents the results of the caregiver screening and assessment process. Chapter Four summarizes the key lessons learned from the initiative. Chapter Five offers recommendations for practice and policy change that will expand and sustain the achievements that were made.

CHAPTER TWO

Methods

This chapter provides details on how the initiative was designed, implemented, and evaluated. We begin by describing the initiative's framework for system change, including the conceptual model, initiative partners, and project organization. Next, we describe the implementation protocols and processes for each component and the strategies undertaken to support implementation. Finally, we present the details of the evaluation plan that guided the initiative's progress and informed the development of the lessons learned and resulting recommendations.

The Initiative's Framework for System Change

The *Helping Families Raise Healthy Children* initiative was designed as a cross-systems quality improvement initiative to change the way local systems work with families facing the related and often co-occurring challenges of parental depression and early childhood developmental delays. The initiative aimed to build new pathways to existing services and expand service options for dual-risk families in a family-centered system that integrated behavioral health screening and care for the caregiver with Part C early intervention services (Figure 2.1). This framework provides opportunities for: (1) screening and improved identification of at-risk families in the Part C early intervention system and maternal and child health care system; (2) enhanced referrals for those identified as being at risk; and (3) access to and support for engagement in relationship-based services in the Part C early intervention and behavioral health systems.

Initiative Partners and Organization

The initiative represents a collaborative effort of more than 35 community partners led by a project team comprising representatives from the initiative's organizing partners (Table 2.1). The three organizing partners (Community Care, The Alliance for Infants and Toddlers, and RAND) and the FAC worked together to implement all aspects of the initiative. Community Care provided the *Helping Families Raise Healthy Children* project director (funded through the grant) to oversee all aspects of the project, including:

- organizing the development of the depression screening and referral protocols
- planning all initiative trainings
- convening a learning collaborative for providers in the early intervention and behavioral health systems
- conducting outreach with initiative partners
- facilitating project team work groups on data collection, policy/outreach, and integration

Figure 2.1
Framework for System Change

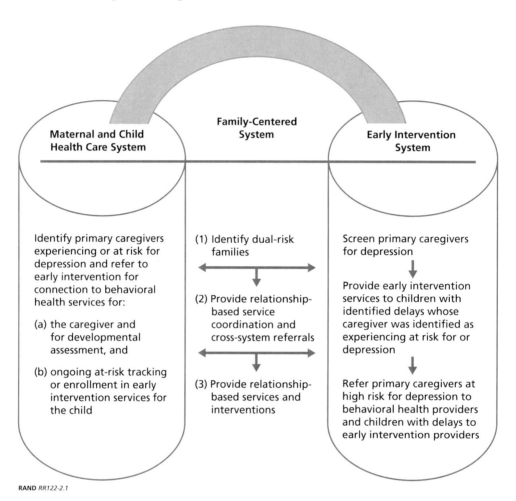

Maternal and Child Health Care System

Family-Centered System

Early Intervention System

Identify primary caregivers experiencing or at risk for depression and refer to early intervention for connection to behavioral health services for:

(a) the caregiver and for developmental assessment, and

(b) ongoing at-risk tracking or enrollment in early intervention services for the child

(1) Identify dual-risk families

(2) Provide relationship-based service coordination and cross-system referrals

(3) Provide relationship-based services and interventions

Screen primary caregivers for depression

Provide early intervention services to children with identified delays whose caregiver was identified as experiencing at risk for or depression

Refer primary caregivers at high risk for depression to behavioral health providers and children with delays to early intervention providers

RAND *RR122-2.1*

- disseminating initiative results and activities at local, state, and national conferences
- preparing grant and funder reports.

Two grant-funded mental health specialists worked at The Alliance to support service coordinators and early intervention providers in their work with screening, referrals, and relationship-based services and treatment. The mental health specialists also managed the cases for families with children whose primary caregivers were identified as experiencing or being at risk for depression but otherwise did not qualify for standard at-risk tracking services or treatment within the Part C early intervention system. The mental health specialists and Alliance clinical director led workshops on relationship-based care for early intervention and behavioral health providers. The grant also provided support for a data manager who was responsible for entering, monitoring, and processing the data collected at The Alliance regarding screening, referrals, and engagement in services. In addition to supporting the development of the screening protocol, referral processes, and cross-system training effort, RAND designed and conducted the evaluation described later in this chapter.

Table 2.1
Initiative Partners

Organizing Partners
Community Care Behavioral Health (grantee)
The Alliance for Infants and Toddlers
RAND Corporation
Family Advisory Council (FAC)

Funders
The Robert Wood Johnson Foundation Local Funding Partnership
The Highmark Foundation (nominating funder)
UPMC Health Plan
The Pittsburgh Foundation
The Fine Foundation
FISA Foundation
Jewish Healthcare Foundation
Pennsylvania Department of Public Welfare, Office of Mental Health and Substance Abuse Services

Community Partners
Part C Early Intervention System
The Alliance for Infants and Toddlers
Early Intervention Network of Service Providers – Achieva, The Early Learning Institute, Integrated Care, Early
Intervention Specialists, Pediatric Therapy Professionals, Therapeutic Early Intervention Services

Maternal and Child Health Care System
Allegheny County, Department of Human Services
Community Care Behavioral Health
Behavioral Health Network of Providers – Allegheny County Department of Human Services Office of Behavioral
Health, Allegheny Family Network, Every Child, Family Resources, Family Services of Western PA, Holy Family
Institute, Matilda Theiss Child Development Center, Mercy Behavioral Health, Mon Yough Community Services,
Re:solve Crisis Network, Sojourner House, Turtle Creek Valley MH/MR
Physical Health Medicaid Managed Care Organizations
Physical Health Providers – Children's Hospital Primary Care Center, KidsPlus Pediatrics, Magee Women's Hospital
of UPMC, Primary Care Health Services Inc., Sto Rox Family Health Center, UPMC Family Medicine

Maternal and Child Health Community Organizations
The Birth Circle
Healthy Start
The Children's Home of Pittsburgh
Perinatal Depression Collaborative
Early Head Start: COTRAIC and Family Foundations
Maternal and Child Health Programs of the Allegheny County Health Department
Family Support Centers
National Fatherhood Initiative

The FAC included eight to ten caregivers experienced with depression or early intervention. The role of the FAC was to ensure the appropriateness and relevance of the training materials and informational materials on depression, inform the development of the screening protocol and referral process, provide feedback on evaluation-related data collection (e.g., the discussion guide for the family interviews), and incorporate a family perspective at cross-system training sessions.

The initiative was supported by a grant from the Robert Wood Johnson Foundation Local Funding Partnerships, and a consortium of local funders, including the Highmark Foundation, UPMC Health Plan, The Pittsburgh Foundation, The Fine Foundation, FISA Foundation, and the Jewish Healthcare Foundation. This project was viewed as a quality improvement initiative in the Medicaid/HealthChoices program in Allegheny County. With the leadership of the Allegheny County Department of Human Services and Community Care, the project obtained additional funds from the Pennsylvania Department of Public Welfare/Office of Mental Health and Substance Abuse Services. Community partners included agencies from the early intervention, behavioral health, physical health care, and community social service systems.

Implementation Protocols and Procedures

The project's implementation involved screening and identifying at-risk families, providing referrals, and supporting engagement in relationship-based services and treatment in the Part C early intervention and behavioral health systems (Figure 2.2). The project's start-up phase (August 2009–January 2010) included development of cross-system practices and protocols for each of these components. These protocols and processes, described below, outline the roles and responsibilities of all participating partners. Throughout implementation, the project team provided technical assistance, infrastructure support, and data collection and communication tools to facilitate interactions within and across systems.

Screening and Identification of At-Risk Families

The first implementation component was to screen and identify at-risk families through three pathways: the screening process, self-identifiers, and community partner referrals.

Families Identified Through the Screening Process

The first pathway involved depression screening for families in Allegheny County who had an infant or toddler with a developmental concern. The screening protocol involved a two-step depression screening process for all new and existing Alliance families. For new families coming into The Alliance for early intervention services, the service coordinators completed the screening process whenever possible during the initial home visit for enrollment in early intervention services. For families already enrolled in early intervention services at the start of the project, the service coordinators conducted screening during their next scheduled visit or evaluation of the family after project implementation. The service coordinator explained to caregivers that, in addition to early intervention services, The Alliance was completing a routine screening process with all of its families that involved questions about how caregivers had been feeling over the past several weeks. The service coordinator then asked the respondents

Figure 2.2
Implementation Components

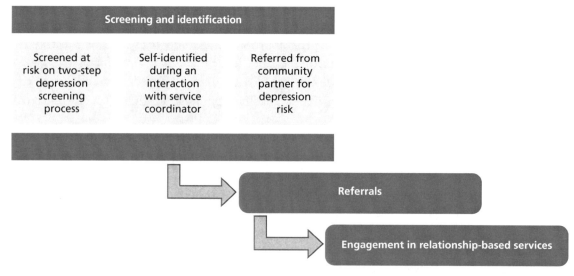

to initial the screening packet if they were willing to have their de-identified information held by RAND. To the extent possible, the service coordinator ensured that the caregiver had some privacy to complete the screening process, which was available in either English or Spanish.

The initial screen consisted of the PHQ-2, a depression screen that is widely used in community health settings (Kroenke, Spitzer, and Williams, 2003). If the caregiver responded positively to either initial screening question, then the nine-question PHQ-9 screen was administered to further assess depressive symptoms (Kroenke, Spitzer, and Williams, 2003). The PHQ-9 is a tool for assisting primary care clinicians in assessing depression that provides a tentative diagnosis and a severity score that aids in selecting and monitoring treatment (MacArthur Initiative on Depression & Primary Care, 2012). Caregivers who scored ten or higher out of 27 on the PHQ-9 were considered to be positive for depression, and the service coordinator explained the result to the caregiver, providing reassurance that there was support available through referrals and access to relationship-based services.

Once a caregiver screened positive for depression, the service coordinator attempted to complete a baseline assessment to evaluate family functioning and provide information about the health of the caregiver and the child. The baseline assessment was designed to help identify the kinds of stressors affecting the caregiver and family and the areas with the greatest need for assistance. The baseline assessment was intended to be completed at the same visit as the screening process or at a later visit, depending on the circumstances. The baseline assessment primarily consisted of the Parenting Stress Index Short Form (PSI-SF), a 36-question survey that is widely used in the field to assess stress in the parent-child relationship (Reitman, Currier, and Stickle, 2002). It also included a series of questions related to the caregiver's health and safety and the child's health.

To monitor changes over time, attempts were made to rescreen all families at six, 12, 18, and 24 months after the baseline screening. Families who screened positive at a follow-up screening received referrals and access to relationship-based services as we will describe later.

Self-Identified Families

The second pathway in the screening and identification component of the initiative involved families who self-identified a need for assistance with caregiver depression during an interaction with their service coordinator at The Alliance. This pathway was not anticipated when the screening protocol described above was initially developed. During implementation, service coordinators noted that some families who did not complete a screen for depression or screened negative self-identified a need for support when the depression screening was offered.

Families Referred by Community Partners

The third pathway involved community-based providers in the maternal and child health care system identifying families with a caregiver at risk for or experiencing depression through screening programs and other efforts. Community-based providers were able to refer these families to The Alliance for developmental assessment and screening for the child, and depression screening and referrals for the caregiver.

Relationship-Based Service Coordination and Referrals

The second component of the initiative was to provide relationship-based service coordination within early intervention and referrals to families who had been identified as at risk for parental depression. The relationship-based service coordination was conceived as a way of engaging with families that recognizes the relationship as the driving factor for most change within the family unit. This approach focuses on supporting the relationship of caregiver and child to enhance delivery and long-term outcomes of early intervention services. While the original plan was to train only interested service coordinators in relationship-based service coordination, ultimately all service coordinators were trained and supported in this approach.

For the referral protocol, when a caregiver screened positive for depression, the Alliance service coordinator explained that all children in the household under the age of three were eligible to have their development monitored, even if they did not qualify for the early intervention services outlined in The Alliance's Individualized Family Service Plan (IFSP) or existing at-risk tracking services. If the family's only risk factor was depression (or another behavioral health concern), then one of the project-funded mental health specialists at The Alliance followed the family, offering more intensive at-risk tracking services. For children who received at-risk tracking services only, the service coordinator followed the family, engaging support from the mental health specialists as needed. For children receiving the early intervention services specified in their IFSPs, the service coordinator also followed the family supported by the mental health specialists as needed.

The referral options included early intervention relationship-based services (e.g., speech therapy, physical therapy), relationship-based behavioral health services (e.g., team-delivered in-home behavioral health services, in-home mobile therapy), other behavioral health services (e.g., outpatient behavioral health therapy), crisis services, and community-based services (e.g., Early Head Start, parenting classes). Caregivers referred for behavioral health services who were evaluated and diagnosed with depression may have received pharmacologic therapy in addition to other services. To determine which referrals might be appropriate, the service coordinator discussed with the caregiver any prior experiences with depression or other behavioral health issues and any treatment received, reviewed assessment responses to discuss the types of stressors the caregiver faces, and assessed whether the family had a support system. Based on this discussion, the service coordinator suggested referral and service options and determined whether the caregiver wanted a referral. If the caregiver declined, the service coordinator provided options for family support, including at-risk tracking by the project's mental health specialist and checked in with the caregiver periodically. If the caregiver accepted a referral, the service coordinator discussed some of the common barriers to accessing behavioral health services and informed the project's mental health specialists about the referral request. For these families, the mental health specialists worked to connect the caregiver and family to the appropriate services and supports. On an ongoing basis, the mental health specialists coordinated services and supports with the service coordinators and with early intervention and community-based providers.

Engagement in Relationship-Based Services

The third component was to provide well-established relationship-based services and therapeutic services within the Part C early intervention and behavioral health systems for caregivers who wished to address their behavioral health issues as well as parenting and the parent-child relationship. The project team selected three dyadic therapies that help parents interpret and respond to their infants' cues, express their own emotions, and prevent or repair damage to the parent-child relationship. These relationship-based interventions met the needs of the target population and, at the same time, aligned with the interests of local service providers in both systems. The project team conducted in-depth training sessions on each relationship-based model, allowing providers to select a model to use. Training was provided for the following therapy models:

- **Promoting First Relationships** emphasizes the importance of attachment between infants/toddlers and their parents/caregivers with a focus on the potentially negative impacts of poverty, family stress, special needs, and behavioral problems on the parent-child relationship (Kelly et al., 2003). The program can be delivered in home or group-based settings and follows a curriculum that uses handouts and videos to strengthen the parent-child relationship.
- **Partners in Parenting Education** aims to promote healthy infant-parent relationships with a focus on developing and maintaining secure attachments between children and caregivers (Dolezol and Butterfield, 1994). The program can be delivered as a home-based intervention, and the curriculum is divided into three parts: Listen, Listen, Listen (e.g., communication skills); Love Is Layers of Sharing (e.g., emotional connections and trust); and Playing Is Learning (e.g., stabilization and socialization). At each session, the provider goes through four phases with the family: Presentation of Concepts; Demonstration; Supervised Parent-Child Interaction; and Evaluation.
- **Nurturing Parenting** (Devall, 2004) was originally developed to prevent and/or treat child abuse and neglect. The program addresses several components of the parent-child relationship, including child development, emotional connections, discipline, communication, and coping with stress. The provider and caregiver work together for the first hour of each visit, and the last half-hour is spent with the parent practicing new skills with coaching when needed. The program can be delivered as a home-based or group-based intervention.

Strategies to Support Initiative Implementation

Throughout implementation, the project team employed a variety of strategies to support the implementation of the initiative components. The strategies were designed to obtain feedback from collaborative partners about the initiative and to continuously improve implementation and the process, individual, and system impact outcomes of the initiative, including conducting cross-system training and education sessions, supporting the screening and referral processes, convening a learning collaborative composed of early intervention and behavioral health providers, conducting outreach to community agencies and partners, and soliciting feedback from initiative partners on the implementation protocols and processes. Each of these areas is described in the following sections.

Conducting Cross-System Provider Training

During the start-up and implementation phases, the project team organized a series of training and education sessions designed to enhance the capacity of local early intervention, behavioral health, and maternal and child health care providers to offer integrated and coordinated service to families with caregivers at risk for or experiencing depression and children at risk for or experiencing developmental delays. Each training session addressed one or more topics related to achieving the initiative's objectives (e.g., caregiver screening/assessment, referrals, and engagement in relationship-based services) and the importance of conducting these activities in a manner that honors and respects family values and priorities and builds trusting relationships with families. The training sessions on relationship-based care used case discussions and examples from culturally diverse families to help explore how families differ in various cultures. Whenever possible, a member of the FAC participated in the training to provide perspective on the training content. To maximize participation for early intervention and behavioral health providers, continuing education credits and partial reimbursement were made available to offset the clinicians' loss of time. Furthermore, a subset of trainings was videotaped and made available for individual viewing online.

Each type of education session is described below:

- **Trainings on the screening protocol and the referral process.** During the start-up phase, the project team developed detailed training materials and conducted training sessions on the use of the initiative's screening tools and referral processes. This training material was provided to service coordinators and supervisors at The Alliance who were expected to play critical start-up roles in depression screening and referral to services and supports. The materials for these trainings were carefully vetted with members of the FAC to ensure their appropriateness and relevance for the target population. Additional training sessions, which were in-depth refreshers on depression, screening procedures, referral processes, and documentation, were provided to service coordinators in Phase 2.
- **Trainings on relationship-based care.** The project team developed and conducted several training sessions that provided information on relationship-based care and models to early intervention and behavioral health providers. The initial training provided an overview of infant mental health and relationship-based care. The subsequent trainings provided more detailed training on the three relationship-based models well-established in the field (Nurturing Parenting, Promoting First Relationships, and Partners in Parenting Education) that were selected for the initiative.

The results of the evaluation for each training session are provided in Appendix A.

Supporting the Screening and Referral Processes

In addition to the training sessions described above, the project team worked to equip Alliance service coordinators and supervisors with the knowledge, tools, resources, and confidence to conduct depression screening and make referrals. The screening protocol included scripts for introducing the screen to caregivers, a list of frequently asked questions, and tips for responding to crisis situations. The project team also developed a resource guide with a complete list of referral options within the community, including eligibility criteria, target populations, and referral processes. This guide was updated periodically and distributed to Alliance service coordinators.

The project-funded mental health specialists played a number of roles. They provided ongoing support and consultation to service coordinators on both the screening and referral processes. They were also available to consult on specific families, accompany the service coordinators on home visits, and provide support when responding to a crisis situation. For the depression screening, the mental health specialists worked with service coordinators to identify challenges (e.g., interviewing skills, comfort level discussing depression) and develop solutions. They also helped service coordinators expand their knowledge of available resources for families in other systems, particularly the behavioral health system for adults, and provided ongoing support related to difficult conversations with families about referrals. Finally, the mental health specialists served as the link between the early intervention service coordinators and the behavioral health providers, providing ongoing support and follow-up assistance to service coordinators and behavioral health providers as needed.

Convening a Learning Collaborative for Providers

To support the integration of relationship-based care into practice, the project team combined providers in the Part C early intervention and behavioral health systems into a group referred to as the "learning collaborative." In the health care arena, the Institute for Healthcare Improvement's *Learning Collaborative Model* and associated *Model for Improvement* involve small multidisciplinary implementation teams from multiple organizations setting aims, choosing simple metrics to determine if a change is helping achieve those aims, and then making an appropriate change (Institute for Healthcare Improvement, 2003). While our approach is consistent with the model's focus on bringing together individuals from across organizations to provide support and share information about overcoming implementation barriers, we did not use metrics to measure change from our group's activities. Our "learning collaborative" was designed to enable providers from the Part C early intervention and behavioral health systems to improve relationship-based practices, share their experiences implementing relationship-based care, and learn from the experiences of others utilizing these practices. Ten meetings or training sessions were held during Phase 2. The early meetings focused on allowing providers who had recently been trained in relationship-based care to discuss their experiences with integrating the relationship-based models into their work with families. Topics included successes and challenges with using the relationship-based techniques, issues related to depression screening, and issues related to coordination across agencies. Learning collaborative participants expressed a desire for continued meetings to reinforce the use of the practices and to continue dialogue and networking across the two systems. Subsequent meetings served dual purposes: Some were devoted to sharing successes and challenges while others were more topic-driven, with presentations on culturally competent engagement skills, infant mental health and attachment, trauma-informed care, and reflective supervision.

Developing Community Partnerships

The project team conducted extensive outreach to existing and new partners in the community who would be identifying and referring families to early intervention based on the caregiver's depression risk. These education and outreach meetings were geared toward partner agency staff members who might be referring families, and provided information and resource materials about depression, its impact on child development, the importance of behavioral health services and treatment, and the referral process. With support from the project team, the community-based agencies could better explain to families why the parent's mental health is important for child development and what early intervention and behavioral health services have to offer. The project team also developed a standard referral form with clear instructions to help facilitate these referrals.

Assessing Progress to Inform Ongoing Implementation

The project team collaborated on a number of activities to engage community partners in the initiative and to solicit their feedback on the initiative protocols and processes, including all-partner meetings, a partner survey, focus groups, and interviews. Two all-partner meetings were conducted during implementation; these were attended by individuals involved in the initiative as implementers, funders, or interested policymakers. Partners were able to reflect on the interim results and early lessons learned from implementation and hear from caregivers and providers about their experiences with various components of the initiative. After the first all-partners meeting, the project team conducted a survey soliciting input about the implementation components, general communication, and collaboration among the partners. The project team reviewed suggestions, organized by topic area, and either noted them as "already addressed" or developed a plan to address the issue, if feasible.

Evaluation Plan

The evaluation plan encompassed a mixed-methods approach, using both quantitative and qualitative data. Three types of measures were used to evaluate the effectiveness of this initiative (Figure 2.3). Process measures helped determine the extent to which the initiative components were being implemented according to plan, thereby providing useful information for potential course corrections during program implementation. System impact measures at the provider and family level offered perspectives on the implementation and system change process, as well as information on changes in provider knowledge, attitudes, beliefs, and behaviors about caregiver depression. Individual outcome measures were assessed at the caregiver level and indicated whether the implementation components (i.e., screening and identification, referrals, and engagement in relationship-based services and treatment) were associated with decreases in depressive symptoms and parenting stress and improvement in caregiver and child health.

During the start-up phase, RAND developed the data collection procedures and protocols described in the next section. Throughout implementation, these procedures and protocols were refined to improve the data collection efforts. We describe the measurement instruments and techniques used to assess process, system impact, and individual outcome measures as well as the data collection procedures and protocols.

Data Collection for Process, Individual Outcome, and System Impact Measures
Process Measures
The process measures span the three components of the initiative: screening and identification, referral, and engagement in services (Figure 2.3). The process measures used to evaluate the screening goals included the number of completed screens, positive screens and assessments, and screening and assessment rates. To evaluate the referral goals, we assessed the number of caregivers referred to services, the referral rate, the number and type of referrals, and the outcome of the referral process. To evaluate the engagement-in-treatment goals, the process measures included the number of referred caregivers engaged in behavioral health treatment as well as the type of treatment, the engagement rate, the number of referred caregivers engaged in relationship-based interventions, and the type of relationship-based interventions.

Individual Outcome Measures
Quantitative data on the outcome measures were collected at the individual level and included the depression screening measures collected on all families at baseline and three follow-up time points (six, 12, and 18 months after baseline). When a caregiver screened positive on the depression screening measure, the assessment information—including measures of parental

Figure 2.3
Process, Individual Outcome, and System Impact Measures

RAND *RR122-2.3*

stress, caregiver health, and child health—were administered at the same time points. The individual-level outcome measures are described in more detail later. The screening and assessment packet is provided in Appendix B.1. Chapter Three lists the results for the baseline and follow-up screenings and assessments conducted from February 2010 through May 2012.

Depression

To assess risk for depression, we used the PHQ-2 as an initial screener and the PHQ-9 for those who screened positive on the PHQ-2 (Kroenke, Spitzer, and Williams, 2003; Kroenke and Spitzer, 2002). Both instruments were self-administered. The PHQ-2 was modified from its original form so that responses were dichotomous (yes/no) rather than asking how often the symptoms occurred. Responding "yes" to either item on the PHQ-2 was considered a positive initial screen, and was followed by a more in-depth assessment with the nine-item instrument. The PHQ-9 includes the two PHQ-2 questions and seven additional questions. The stem question is, "Over the last 2 weeks, how often have you been bothered by any of the following problems?" The two items in both screens are "little interest or pleasure in doing things," and "feeling down, depressed, or hopeless." The two items were asked again in the PHQ-9 with the PHQ-9 response options of "not at all," "several days," "more than half the days," and "nearly every day," scored as 0, 1, 2, and 3, respectively. Other questions focus on sleep, appetite, concentration, and suicidal feelings. The PHQ-9 has a maximum score of 27; a cutoff score of ten was used to identify those caregivers at high risk for depression, with a score of ten to 14 indicating a provisional diagnosis of minor depression. According to the scoring guidelines, a score of 15–19 indicates a provisional diagnosis of moderately severe major depression and a score of 20 or more indicates a provisional diagnosis of severe major depression (MacArthur Initiative on Depression and Primary Care, 2012). The PHQ-2 and PHQ-9 have shown strong sensitivity and specificity for detecting depression in both general and in low-income populations (Arroll et al., 2010; Cutler et al., 2007), and have comparable performance to lengthier depression screens commonly used in primary care settings (Flynn et al., 2011; Kroenke et al., 2010).

Parental Stress

We used the PSI-SF to examine parental stress (Reitman, Currier, and Stickle, 2002). This is a 36-item measure derived from the longer Parenting Stress Index (PSI) that has demonstrated good sensitivity to change in prevention and intervention programs aimed at low-income women with depression or other psychosocial problems (Browne and Talmi, 2005; Cowen, 1998). The PSI-SF has three subscales: parental distress, parent-child dysfunctional interaction, and difficult child characteristics. Each subscale contains 12 items. Caregivers rated their level of agreement—5 (strongly agree) to 1 (strongly disagree)—with statements about themselves or feelings about/interactions with their child (e.g., "I often have the feeling that I cannot handle things very well," and "My child rarely does things for me that make me feel good"). In prior research, the subscales have shown good internal consistency, with Cronbach's alphas of .87 for the parental distress scale, .80 for the parent-child dysfunctional interaction scale, .85 for the difficult child scale, and .91 for the total stress scale (Abidin, 1995). We computed a score for each subscale as well as a total score, with higher scores indicating more stress for each dimension. We also identified those in our sample whose scores fell within the "clinical" range for each subscale and for total stress (Reitman, Currier, and Stickle, 2002).

Caregiver Health and Safety

To assess caregiver health, we incorporated select questions about general health status, sleep, diet, exercise, preventive health care, and emergency room visits from the Behavioral Risk Factor Surveillance System, the National Health and Nutrition Examination Survey, and the National Health Interview Survey (NHIS) (see Table 2.2). To assess caregiver safety, we also included a question about whether the caregiver was in an unsafe relationship. This question is used by the medical advocates for the local women's shelter use to screen for intimate partner violence in local emergency rooms.

Child Health

To assess child health, we incorporated questions drawn from the NHIS about emergency room visits ("During the past six months, how many times has your child gone to a hospital emergency room about his/her health? This includes emergency room visits that resulted in a hospital admission"), preventive health care ("Does the child have a physician that he/she sees regularly?"), and immunizations ("Based on the American Academy of Pediatric Standards, are the child's immunizations up to date?").

System Impact Measures

We assessed system impact at the provider (early intervention and behavioral health) and caregiver levels with qualitative data collected through focus groups, training surveys, and telephone interviews.

Table 2.2
Caregiver Health and Safety Items

Item	Response Options
Would you say that in general your health is...?	• Excellent • Very good • Good • Fair • Poor
During the past 30 days, for about how many days have you felt you did not get enough rest or sleep?	# of Days
In general, how healthy is your overall diet? Would you say...?	• Excellent • Very good • Good • Fair • Poor
During the past month, did you participate in any physical activities or exercises such as running, calisthenics, golf, gardening, or walking for exercise?	• Yes • No
What kind of place do you USUALLY go when you need routine or preventive care, such as a physical examination or check-up?	• Doesn't get preventive care anywhere • Clinic or health center • Doctor's office or HMO • Hospital emergency room • Hospital outpatient department • Some other place • Doesn't go to one place most often
During the past six months, how many times have you gone to a hospital emergency room about your own health (This includes emergency room visits that resulted in a hospital admission)?	# of times
Are you currently in a relationship that is not safe?	• Yes • No

Early Intervention and Behavioral Health Providers

To obtain feedback from key stakeholders on implementation and the system-change process, RAND met with three groups of early intervention and behavioral health providers and two groups of service coordinators to hear their views and suggestions on implementation of the initiative and to enable ongoing quality improvement. With the early intervention and behavioral health providers, RAND developed a discussion guide focused on the referral process, the initiative trainings on relationship-based care, using relationship-based approaches in working with families, the learning collaborative, and communication and coordination with providers in other systems (Appendix B.2). The service coordinator group's protocol was designed to elicit feedback on the ease or difficulty of administering the depression screen, the ideal timing of the depression screen, the overall approach to integrating the screening protocol into routine practice in the Part C early intervention system, and the referral process (Appendix B.3).

For early intervention and behavioral health providers, we also conducted a training evaluation with measures designed to obtain information on changes in knowledge, attitudes, beliefs, and behaviors (i.e., screening, referral, and treatment) related to caregiver depression and relationship-based care. Data collection for the training evaluation included pre- and post-training surveys at each initiative training session. The early sessions focused on training Alliance service coordinators and supervisors on the screening/assessment process and the referral process. These trainings had 109 participants; 101 of them completed the training survey. Following the overview training, separate training sessions were conducted for each of the three relationship-based intervention models. These had 414 participants, with 292 completing the training survey. For all training sessions, surveys were administered before the session began and immediately following its completion. Participant information, such as area of expertise, was collected in the pre-training materials. Several measures were administered in both the pre- and post-training surveys, including measures of knowledge, confidence in implementing skills or techniques relevant to the training, comfort in performing tasks relevant to the training, and, in some cases, attitudes toward evidence-based practices.

Many of the system impact measures included on the training surveys were developed specifically for this initiative and tailored to the content. The items on the pre- and post-training surveys were relevant to the training and designed to measure participants' knowledge, confidence in implementing skills or techniques, and comfort in performing tasks. Many of the surveys also included a measure of attitudes toward evidence-based practices. The Evidence-Based Practice Attitudes Scale (Aarons, 2004) is a previously developed instrument that was employed in multiple training sessions of the initiative to assess attitudes toward using evidence-based therapies and interventions. This scale includes items that address four subscales: requirements ("... How likely would you be to adopt [the technique] if it was required by your supervisor?"), appeal ("...How likely would you be to adopt [the technique] if it was intuitively appealing?"), openness ("I am willing to try new types of therapy/interventions even if I have to follow a treatment manual"), and divergence ("I would not use manualized therapy/interventions"). Items are rated on a scale of 1 (not at all) to 5 (to a very great extent). Appendix A provides details of training participation and the results of the training evaluation activities. Overall, the training sessions were well received and effective at increasing knowledge of the effects of maternal depression on the early development of the brain, infant-caregiver attachment, and relationship-based care.

Caregivers

In an effort to obtain feedback from those served by The Alliance, RAND conducted 15 telephone interviews with caregivers who had a range of experiences related to the initiative components of screening, referral, and treatment. For these family interviews, RAND project team members developed the interview discussion guide in consultation with the other members of the project team and the FAC, and conducted practice interviews with FAC members. Based on their feedback, the RAND project team members modified the family interview discussion guide. Most changes involved streamlining the interview process to lessen the burden of time on caregivers, and to enhance caregiver comfort in speaking about their experiences with screening, referral and treatment engagement. The final discussion guide focused on the initiative's screening and identification, referral, and engagement-in-services components (Appendix B.4).

Data Collection Activities

All data collection activities were approved by the RAND Human Subjects Protection Committee. Community Care and The Alliance shared de-identified data with RAND for the purposes of the evaluation.

Quantitative Data

Data related to screening were recorded on a Screening/Assessment Tracking Form completed for each family by the service coordinator (Appendix B.5). All materials were provided in Spanish for Spanish-speaking caregivers. When necessary, translators accompanied the service coordinator on the home visit to conduct the screening and assessment in the native language. Once the screening/assessment packet had been completed, the service coordinator submitted the packet to the data manager at The Alliance, who then recorded the information on a Screening Assessment Tracking From and entered the data in the project database. The data manager also updated the form and database with subsequent screening or assessment activity. The project's mental health specialists initiated meetings with Alliance supervisors to provide feedback on screening rates for individual service coordinators. This strategy helped to identify service coordinators with lower screening rates so that further support could be provided to ensure that the service coordinators understood the screening protocol and were comfortable administering it.

For caregivers who screened positive, Alliance service coordinators completed assessments of parenting stress, caregiver health and safety, and child health. Because of time constraints, these assessments were often not completed during the same visit. In an effort to improve the assessment completion rate, the project's mental health specialists began attending monthly staff meetings at The Alliance to discuss the importance of completing the assessment portion of the process. At these meetings, the service coordinators were reminded that the assessment provides information about a family's needs and can help drive decisionmaking about referrals.

For the follow-up assessments, the data manager initially distributed new screening packets to the service coordinator approximately one month prior to the follow-up due date. This was intended to serve as a reminder for the service coordinator to complete the screen on the next family visit. However, this process did not work well because the packets were not directly placed in the family's file and the service coordinator did not always have the packet when visiting the family. The process was revised so that the data manager generated the new screening packet when entering the initial screening information. If the caregiver scored positive or requested services on a previous screen, the data manager would attach a note to the new packet reminding the service coordinator to administer the entire assessment packet at follow-up, regardless of the follow-up screening score. The data manager would then give the packet to the service coordinator, who placed it in the family's file to take on the next visit. In an attempt to improve the follow-up screening and assessment rate, the initiative provided $5 grocery store gift cards to service coordinators for each completed follow-up assessment during the last year of data collection..

For families with a caregiver who screened positive or who requested a referral, data were collected on a Referral Tracking Form (Appendix B.6). The service coordinators and mental health specialists completed and updated these forms as necessary with information on the referral outcome. This information on engagement in services was obtained through contacts with the early intervention and behavioral health providers to whom the families were referred. Periodically, the data manager asked the service coordinators and mental health specialists to provide updates on known service receipt.

For referred caregivers on Medical Assistance, data were tracked on claims paid by Community Care for behavioral health treatment rendered by behavioral health providers in its network. These data were used to measure whether caregivers who had been referred for services initiated behavioral health treatment, the diagnosis recorded at the onset of services, the timing of their engagement in services in relation to being screened, the number of times they received behavioral health services, and the types of behavioral health services received.

Qualitative Data
The qualitative data collection for the system impact measures included focus groups, family interviews, and training surveys.

- Focus Groups: Data were collected from three groups of early intervention and behavioral health providers during April 2011 and two groups of service coordinators during July and August 2011. Each group had six to 12 participants.
- Family Interviews: During January and February 2012, RAND researchers spoke with 15 individual caregivers about their experiences and asked them to discuss what aspects of the process worked well for them, as well as areas needing improvement. Although experiences varied across families, particularly depending on how they were identified for referrals, most caregivers were willing to speak openly about their experiences. The perspectives shared during the family interviews helped inform the results and lessons learned.
- Training Surveys: At each initiative training session, surveys were administered before the session began and immediately following its completion to assess changes in knowledge, attitudes, beliefs, and behaviors (i.e., screening, referral, and engagement in treatment) related to relationship-based care. Overall, the training surveys targeted the 109 participants in the screening and referral process training sessions and the 414 participants in the relationship-based intervention model training sessions (Appendix A).

Data Analysis

The analytic plan examined the process, system impact, and individual outcome measures for the entire data collection period (February 2010 through May 2012), as well as by phase. This approach enabled the project team to use the results and lessons learned from Phase 1 implementation (February 2010–January 2011) to inform the Phase 2 implementation (February 2011–May 2012).

Quantitative Data

The quantitative analyses (descriptive frequencies, means, standard deviations) and bivariate statistics (chi-square, t-tests, analysis of variance) describe the outcomes of the individual outcome measures. The significance tests were conducted to examine differences when the sample size was at least 20 per group. Since this evaluation was designed to inform implementation processes for the initiative and usual care within early intervention was enhanced through the initiative, a comparison group of families who did not receive any services was not feasible. The analysis of individual outcomes examined indicators at baseline and evaluated changes in outcomes over time for those caregivers served by the initiative.

Qualitative Data

The qualitative data analysis of the results of the focus groups, training surveys, and telephone interview findings informed the development of the factors affecting implementation. After completing the qualitative data collection, we synthesized information for the results section of this report. In identifying the factors that facilitated or hindered implementation, we reviewed the relevant findings from the focus group and telephone interview summaries, as well as the training survey results. For example, in examining the referral processes, we carefully reviewed the summary notes of the provider focus groups and caregiver interviews. This analysis revealed the factors that facilitated the referral process, the challenges in the referral process, and the strategies used to address the challenges.

CHAPTER THREE

Results

This chapter focuses on our evaluation of the implementation process, system impact, and individual-level outcome measures for the *Helping Families Raise Healthy Children* initiative (Figure 3.1). Data collection was conducted over a 28-month period from February 2010 through May 2012. We begin by presenting the results of our assessment of implementation, organized by the process measures for the three components of the initiative (i.e., screening and identification, referral, and engagement in services) with a focus on the screening, referral, and engagement rates (Section A). Next, we summarize the results of our system impact measures, which assessed factors affecting implementation of each of the three initiative components and provided perspectives on the successes and challenges in the system change process (Section B). Finally, we describe the results of the individual-level outcome measures at baseline and follow-up, including depression, parental stress, and caregiver and child health and safety

Figure 3.1
Summary Screening, Referral, and Engagement Rates from Maternal Depression Literature

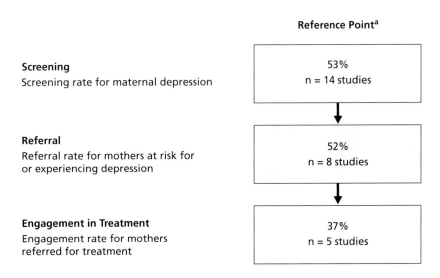

[a] The reference points represent rates found in the literature for similar at-risk populations (e.g., screening: Armstrong and Small, 2007; Garcia, LaCaze, and Ratanasen, 2011; LaRocco-Cockburn et al., 2003; referral: Chaudron et al., 2004; Sheeder, Kabir, and Stafford, 2009; Yonkers et al., 2009; and engagement: Miranda et al., 2003; Smith et al., 2009).
RAND *RR122-3.1*

(Section C). The linkage between the process and individual-level outcome measures is shown in the figure in Appendix C.

Section A. Assessment of the Implementation Process: Screening and Identification, Referral, and Engagement in Services

To support its aims, the initiative implemented processes for screening and identification of at-risk families, referrals, and engagement in relationship-based services in the Part C early intervention and behavioral health systems.

In order to determine markers for improvement in these processes, we summarized reference points from descriptive, intervention, and quality improvement studies reporting rates of depression screening, referral, and engagement for at-risk populations. To ensure reference rates were meaningful for the initiative, we included studies that focused on low-income (and often minority) mothers, rather than including studies that focused on general populations of mothers or women. We established reference points by calculating the mean rates of screening, referral, and engagement in treatment across studies. Figure 3.2 presents a summary of the reference points used to mark improvement in depression screening, referrals for behavioral health services, and engagement in services. Details of the reference studies are include in Appendix D.

Depression Screening Rates. Survey estimates of maternal depression screening indicate an average screening rate of 53 percent (e.g., Armstrong and Small, 2007; Garcia, LaCaze, and Ratanasen, 2011; LaRocco-Cockburn et al., 2003; Seehusen et al., 2005; Segre et al., 2011),

Figure 3.2
Key Components of the Initiative

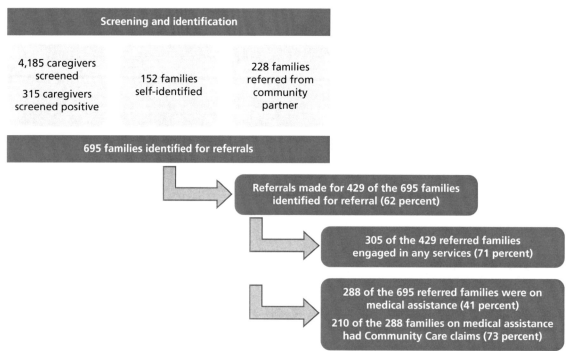

with estimates as low as 8 percent in community pediatric primary care (Olson et al., 2002), and as high as 67 percent by obstetricians in academic medical settings (Gordon, et al., 2006). Recent reports from Pennsylvania's Office of Medical Assistance Programs indicate that rates of prenatal ranged from 51 percent in 2008 to 65 percent in 2009 (OMAP 2008; OMAP, 2009), and postpartum depression screening rates ranged from 34 percent in 2008 to 51 percent in 2009. However, these rates do not distinguish physicians using validated screening tools from those who rely on non-standardized screening methods, and they represent both perinatal and postnatal depression. While this literature may provide the most useful references in the absence of literature about caregivers of children requiring early intervention services, these studies reference a potentially distinct population (e.g., the cause of depression may differ, or presence of child developmental delays may differ).

Referral rates. Survey estimates of referral rates following a positive depression screen typically average 52 percent (e.g., Chaudron et al., 2004; Sheeder, Kabir, and Stafford, 2009; Yonkers et al., 2009). In most studies, "referral" was not explicitly defined but typically reflected the participant/patient receiving a recommendation for a specific provider or service. Rates vary considerably by setting and by available follow-up services. Reports of referrals in publicly funded obstetrics or primary care health clinics tend to represent the lower range of referral rates (e.g., Olson et al., 2005; Yonkers et al., 2009), whereas referrals from pediatric clinics in large, academic settings have been higher, around 50 percent (Chaudron et al., 2004). Such differences may also reflect differences in collaborative communication with mental health services or preexisting systems in place to facilitate referrals.

Engagement in treatment rates. Studies of low-income women reported an average baseline engagement rate (participation in at least one session) of approximately 37 percent for depressed women (e.g., Miranda et al., 2003; Sit et al., 2009; Smith et al., 2009; Wiggins et al., 2005); engagement in multiple sessions (i.e., more than one session) is typically lower, ranging from 6 to 17 percent (Smith et al., 2009; Miranda et al., 2003). Generally, the literature shows that engagement rates vary with types of services offered; e.g., 94 percent for home visits and 16 percent for onsite community mental health care (Wiggins et al., 2005; Sit et al., 2009). Moreover, the definition of engagement varies broadly, as do the terms used (e.g., engaged, enrolled, participated).

In this section, we describe the results of implementation of the three initiative components (Figure 3.3) and compare the screening, referral, and engagement-in-services rates with the reference points derived from our review of the literature (Figure 3.4; also see Appendix D for details about comparison studies).

Screening and Identification Results

As described in the previous chapter, the initiative's screening and identification component offered multiple pathways for identifying at-risk families and providing them with referrals. While it was expected that most families would be identified through a positive score on the depression screen, a majority of families came through the other two channels. Details for each pathway are described below.

Families Identified Through the Screening Process

The first pathway was families screened and identified through the newly established depression screening process at The Alliance. Following the initiative protocol, service coordinators at The Alliance attempted to screen caregivers from all new families referred to them for child-level early intervention developmental screening and assessment. During the 28-month data collection period, service coordinators completed screenings with 4,185 families.

The overall screening rate for new families to The Alliance was 63 percent. The screening rate was calculated by dividing the total number of completed screens for families new to The Alliance (n=3,647) by the total number of initial home visits with new families (n=5,789) during the period. Project benchmarks were to screen 70 percent of families by the end of the first year of data collection (February 2010–January 2011) and 90 percent of families by the end of the project (February 2011–May 2012). Throughout the data collection period, a number of strategies were implemented in an attempt to improve the overall screening rate, including systematically tracking initial home visits and following up with service coordinators and supervisors during regular staff meetings. Nonetheless, high caseloads among service coordinators and heavy workloads during the initial home visits contributed to screening rates that were lower than expected.

While falling below the target, the screening rate of 63 percent generally exceeds average screening rates found in other descriptive, intervention, and quality improvement studies (see Appendix D, Table D.1). The initiative's efforts to select an appropriate validated screening tool, integrate the screening protocol with existing procedures, train service coordinators on the screening tool and protocol, and provide ongoing support to the service coordinators all contributed to an overall screening rate higher than the average of these reference points.

After an initial rise in depression screens at the beginning of the project as service coordinators screened both new and existing families, the number of screens largely stabilized at an average of 149 screens per month for the full data collection period (Figure 3.3).

Completed screens were conducted with both new and existing families with some variation in case type (Figure 3.4). Among new families, the vast majority of screens (83 percent) were for families with IFSPs, indicating that the child had one or more developmental delays.

Figure 3.3
Completed Screens by Month (n=4,185)

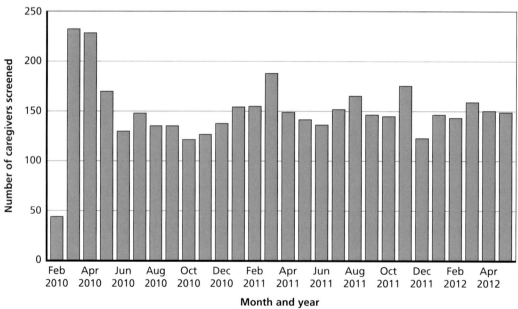

Figure 3.4
Completed Screens by Case Type (n=4,185)

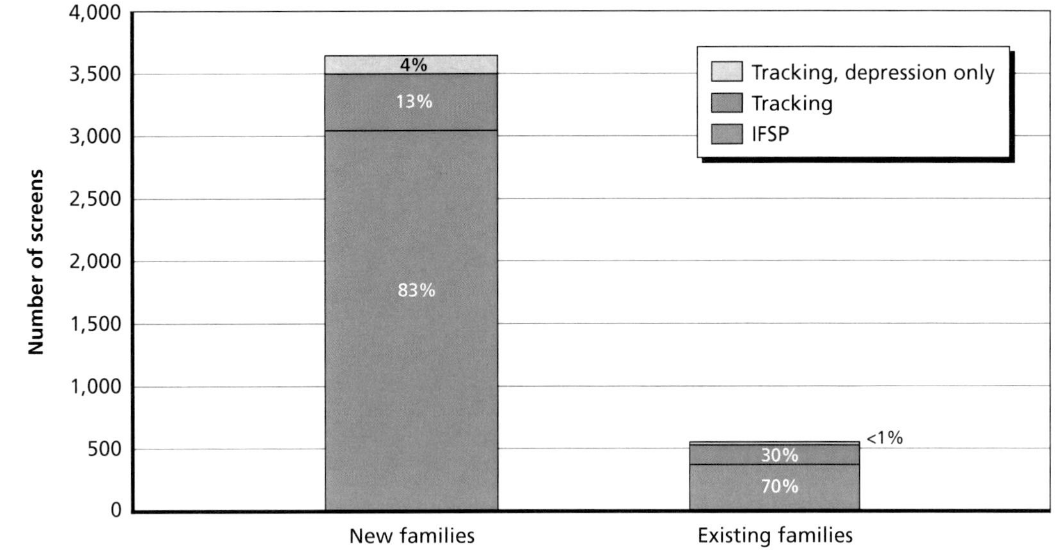

RAND *RR122-3.4*

Thirteen percent of screened families were in The Alliance's tracking group for children at risk for developmental delays. The remaining 4 percent of new families were those who had been recognized by community-based partners as at risk for or experiencing depression and referred to The Alliance for at-risk tracking services based on the caregiver's depression risk. For existing families (those already involved with The Alliance when implementation began), the completed screens occurred more frequently among IFSP families, with whom Alliance service coordinators typically had more contact.

The initial screens were completed by Alliance service coordinators on different types of home visits with the families (Figure 3.5). While 86 percent of the screens were completed at the initial home visit following the initiative protocol, 5 percent were conducted at a follow-up visit and 9 percent at some other visit. This variation reflects the flexibility of the screening protocol that allowed service coordinators to complete the depression screen when it fit best with the caregiver's needs and plans for the visit.

As shown in Table 3.1, the vast majority of caregivers screened were female (97 percent) and the birth parent of the child (99 percent). Approximately two-thirds of the children of screened caregivers were male, with ages distributed evenly across the age categories served by The Alliance. Two-thirds of the children were white (66 percent), and about a fifth were African-American (22 percent).

Of the 4,185 caregivers screened, 315 were identified for the referral component through this screening process (Figure 3.2).

Self-Identified Families

The second pathway in the screening and identification component of the initiative involved families who self-identified a need for assistance with caregiver depression during an interaction with their service coordinator. These families declined to complete a depression screen or screened negative for depression but self-identified a need for support during a visit with their

Figure 3.5
Screenings by Visit Type (n=4,185)

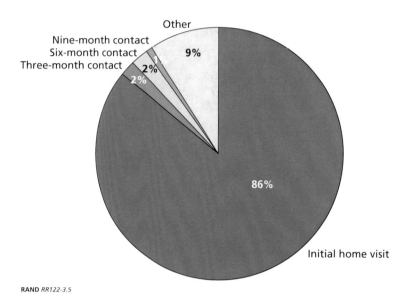

service coordinator. While this pathway was not anticipated when developing the screening and referral protocols, the processes were modified to enable service coordinators to refer caregivers to behavioral health and other services. The service coordinators found that discussing how the caregiver feels, looking at their emotional status through the lens of infant/toddler development, and offering a depression screen could create an opening for offering support. This dialogue allows caregivers to self-identify a need for services. A total of 152 families were identified for referrals via this pathway.

Families Recognized by Community Partners

The third pathway included families with a caregiver at risk for or experiencing depression who were identified through screening programs and other efforts by community-based providers in the maternal and child health care system. These families were referred to The Alliance for relationship-based service coordination and referrals even though their children had not been identified as experiencing a developmental delay. Once referred, The Alliance conducted a developmental screening and evaluation to determine eligibility for early intervention services and for the relationship-based service coordination and referrals offered through the initiative. A referral form with clear instructions that could be faxed to The Alliance was created to help facilitate this process.

To engage the maternal and child health care system in making referrals to early intervention based on the caregiver's depression risk, the initiative conducted outreach activities with providers, practices, and agencies within the maternal and child health care system to describe the initiative, establish relationships with agencies and organizations, and explain the referral process. These meetings, held for staff members at the community-based agencies who might be referring families, provided information and resource materials about depression, its impact on child development, the importance of behavioral health services and treatment, and the referral process. The education and outreach efforts focused on physical health providers, including pediatric, obstetrics and gynecology, and family medicine practices likely to come

Table 3.1
Caregiver and Child Information

Caregiver Information	Percentage (n=4,185)
Caregiver gender	
Female	97
Male	3
Caregiver relationship to child	
Birth parent	99
Adoptive parent	1
Grandparent	1
Other	<1
Child information	
Child gender	Percentage (n=4,179)
Female	37
Male	63
Child age	Percentage (n=4,179)
Less than 1	42
1	30
2	28
Child race/ethnicity	Percentage (n=3,529)
White (non-Hispanic)	66
African American (non-Hispanic)	22
Hispanic	2
Asian	3
Other or biracial	8

NOTE: Percentages do not total 100 due to rounding.

into contact with parents of infants and toddlers, nurse home-visiting programs, early childhood programs such as Healthy Start, and other community-based agencies and organizations.

A total of 228 new families were referred to The Alliance through this pathway. The highest percentage of these referrals (46 percent) came from physical health providers, including pediatric, obstetrics and gynecology, and family medicine practices (Table 3.2). The Health Department's Nurse Family Partnership program also identified and referred families to The Alliance (19 percent), as did the Birth Circle doula program (11 percent), Healthy Start

Table 3.2
Referral Source for Families Identified by Community-Based Providers

Referral Source	Percentage of Families (n=228)
Physical health provider	46
Health Department	19
The Birth Circle	11
Healthy Start	8
Behavioral health provider	3
Family Support Center	1
Other	13

(8 percent), and other community-based providers. Eighteen percent of these families needed an IFSP to address the child's developmental delays. These represent children with developmental delays who may not otherwise have been identified for early intervention services.

Referral Results
Families Identified for Referrals

From the three screening and identification pathways described above, a total of 695 families were identified for the referral process as a result of the caregiver's mental health. Families were distributed across all pathways (Table 3.3), including depression screening at The Alliance (45 percent), self-identification (22 percent), and referrals from community partners (33 percent).

The 695 caregivers who were identified for referrals had a variety of needs or issues based on their current situation and history (Figure 3.6). These data likely underestimate the percentage of caregivers experiencing these needs because of an inability to distinguish caregivers who indicated they did not have the identified need or issue from caregivers who did not provide information about their needs. Of all these caregivers, one-quarter indicated that they were pregnant or had an infant less than six months of age. Nearly one-fifth of caregivers (19 percent) had a transportation-related need, and approximately one-fifth (17 percent) indicated that they had a previously diagnosed mental health disorder. Eight percent of the caregivers identified a history of domestic violence, 7 percent had some current or past drug involvement, and 5 percent had a history of alcohol use or abuse. One-quarter of caregivers (25 percent) identified other needs or issues, including caregiver depression, physical health problems, and problems with housing, among others.

These caregivers also had current or prior needs for behavioral health services. More than one-half of caregivers (53 percent) identified for family-centered care and service coordination indicated that they wanted a referral for behavioral health services (Figure 3.7). Just under one-quarter (22 percent) had received behavioral health services previously. Ten percent indicated that they were receiving behavioral health services at the time of the referral(s).

There were some differences in family demographic characteristics by pathway for the families identified for referrals (Table 3.4). The characteristics were similar for the "screened positive" and "self-identified" pathways. This is not unexpected, because the families identified through these two pathways were both already involved with early intervention and reflected the early intervention population. For those referred by community partners, there was an even distribution across boys and girls, whereas for the other pathways there were significantly more boys than girls. The children referred by community partners were also significantly younger, with a higher percentage of children under one year of age; and there was a much higher percentage of African-Americans here than in the other pathways.

Table 3.3
Pathway for Families Referred for Services

Pathway	Percentage of Families (n=695)
Screening at The Alliance	45
Self-identified	22
Referral from community partner	33

**Figure 3.6
Caregiver Needs/Issues (n=695)**

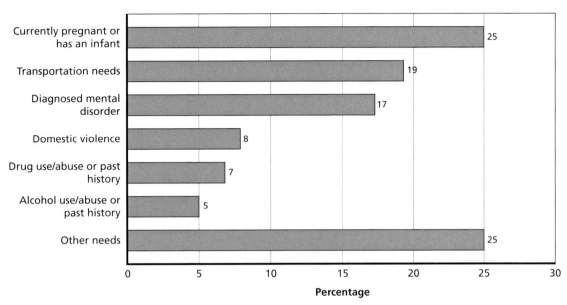

**Figure 3.7
Caregiver Behavioral Health Services (n=695)**

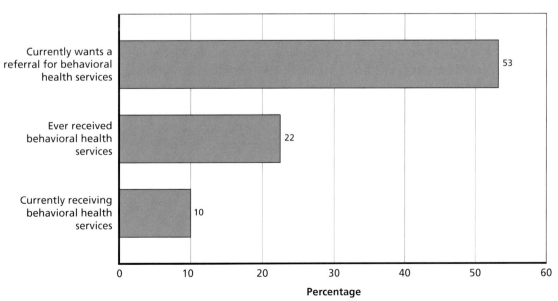

Table 3.4
Family Demographic Characteristics by Referral Pathway

Demographic	Screened Positive (by percentage, n=315)	Self-Identified (by percentage, n=152)	Referred by Community Partner (by percentage, n=228)	Significance Level (chi-square test)
Caregiver gender				NA*
Male	2	4	1	
Female	98	96	99	
Child gender				p<.05
Male	63	59	51	
Female	37	41	49	
Child age				p<.01
Under 1	36	45	81	
1–2 years	32	33	12	
2–3 years	32	23	7	
Child race				p<.01
African American	34	35	55	
White	49	47	22	
Other	17	20	23	
Received medical assistance				n.s.
Yes	74	79	80	
No	26	21	20	

NOTE: Percentages do not total 100 across pathways due to rounding.

* NA = not applicable. Chi–square comparison test not run because of cell sizes of less than 5.

n.s. = nonsignificant

Referral Rate

For all caregivers identified through one of the pathways, the service coordinator and caregiver discussed any prior experiences with depression or other behavioral health issues, any treatment or services received, the types of stressors the caregiver faced, and whether the family had a support system. Based on this discussion, the service coordinator then suggested referral and service options based on the guide developed by the project team and the relationships they had developed with providers during training and networking opportunities. If the caregiver declined a referral, the service coordinator provided options for family support, including at-risk tracking by the grant-funded mental health specialist, and checked in with the caregiver periodically. If the caregiver accepted, the service coordinator discussed some of the common barriers to accessing services, completed a referral form, and informed the project's mental health specialists. The mental health specialists then worked toward connecting the caregiver and family to the appropriate services and supports.

Referrals were made for 429 of the 695 families identified, a rate of 62 percent. The referral rate was calculated by dividing the number of families referred by the number of positive screens or caregivers who requested services. For some of the 266 families who did not receive a referral, service coordinators provided information on the reason why a referral was not made. Nearly one-fifth (19 percent) of these families were discharged, or The Alliance lost contact with them before any referrals were made. Another 18 percent declined services before the referral was made. Referrals were not made for 26 percent because the caregiver indicated they were already receiving services. For the remaining 37 percent of those not referred, the service coordinator did not provide information about the reason.

Referral rates varied somewhat according to the pathway through which caregivers were identified as needing referrals (Figure 3.8). Among families identified through the screening process at The Alliance (n=315), 59 percent received a referral. For caregiver-initiated requests (n=152), 88 percent received a referral indicating that a small percentage of those who had identified a need for support did not receive a referral. Some of these families may have been discharged from The Alliance before a referral was made. Among caregivers identified by community partners (n=228), 48 percent received a referral. The higher referral rates among families already receiving services at The Alliance likely reflect the already established interaction between caregivers and service coordinators. The families referred by community-based partners were new to The Alliance and the relationships had not yet developed to the point where caregivers were accepting of referrals or the families were difficult to reach so referrals could not be made.

Overall, referral rates for the initiative were comparable to or exceeded an average of 52 percent seen for comparable target populations for studies in the maternal depression literature (e.g., Chaudron et al., 2004; Sheeder, Kabir, and Stafford, 2009; Yonkers et al., 2009). (See Appendix D, Table D.2.) For the *Helping Families Raise Healthy Children* initiative, efforts such as cross-system meetings, collaborative development of referral processes, training and support for early intervention service coordinators, and a learning collaborative that brought together early intervention and behavioral health providers helped improve communication and coordination to ensure that appropriate referrals were made.

Figure 3.8
Referral Rate by Pathway

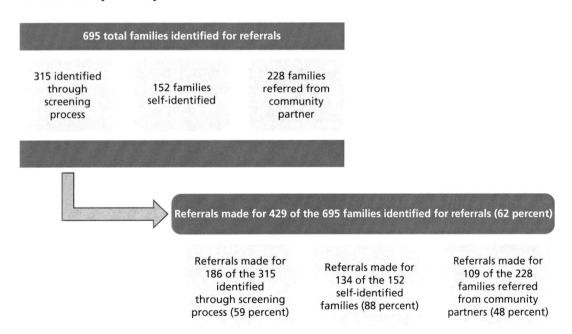

RAND *RR122-3.8*

Referral Types

Families were referred to a variety of services using the initiative's referral protocol (Figure 3.9). Nearly one-half of the 429 referred families (43 percent) were referred to one of the early intervention providers trained by the initiative in relationship-based care. Families were also referred to the behavioral health providers who had been trained in relationship-based approaches: 30 percent received a referral to team-delivered, in-home behavioral health services, and 25 percent for in-home mobile therapy. Together, 87 percent were referred to one of the three in-home service options (i.e., early intervention relationship-based services, team-delivered in-home behavioral health services, or in-home mobile therapy). Sixteen percent were referred for community-based services such as Early Head Start, parenting classes, and Family Support Centers.

Engagement-in-Services Results

Engagement Among All Caregivers

Engagement Rate

According to information gathered by Alliance service coordinators or mental health specialists from providers on referral outcomes, a total of 305 of the 429 caregivers who were referred engaged in services. This total included caregivers who received Medical Assistance and were eligible for services through Community Care (58 percent), or had private insurance (12 percent). The remaining caregivers who engaged in services did not have insurance or did not provide insurance information.

Overall, the engagement rate for caregivers who received at least one referral was 71 percent. Caregivers were counted as having engaged in services if the family had received at least one session of one of the services for which they received a referral. The engagement rate was

Figure 3.9
Referral Types (n=429)

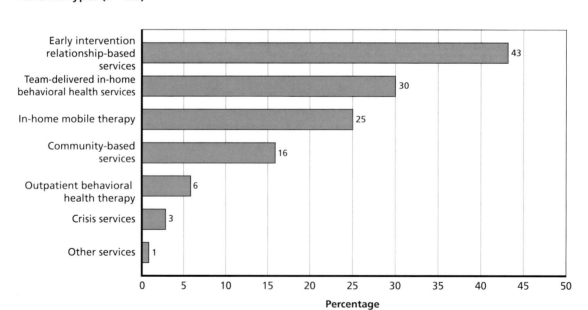

NOTE: Percentages add up to more than 100 because families could receive more than one referral.
RAND RR122-3.9

calculated by dividing the number of families who attended one or more such sessions by the total number of referrals. The relatively liberal definition of engagement was necessary because of limitations in the ability to collect data on referral outcomes. The Alliance attempted to confirm whether each referred family had received any services, but was unable to determine the number of sessions received. While a limitation, this definition of engagement is comparable to how other descriptive, intervention, and quality improvement studies report processes following referrals (e.g., initiation of services or treatment, completion of first visit). (See Table D.3 in Appendix D.)

Engagement rates were consistent across the pathways through which caregivers were identified (Figure 3.10). Among families identified through the screening process at The Alliance (n=186), 67 percent of caregivers engaged in one or more services to which they were referred. For self-identified caregivers (n=134), 75 percent engaged in services, and among caregivers identified by community partners (n=109), 73 percent engaged in services.

At the end of the first year of implementation, the project-funded mental health specialists began to systematically track engagement and follow-up with both families and providers to ensure that referred families engaged in services. Among those families who did not engage in services, common explanations for lack of engagement or lack of information about engagement included (1) the family had been discharged because the child was over the age of three or because The Alliance no longer had valid contact information for the family, (2) the family declined to participate in services or did not follow through with scheduled appointments, and (3) the referral agency could not reach the family.

Compared to an average engagement rate of 37 percent across studies with comparable populations (see Appendix D, Table D.3), the 71 percent engagement rate for the initiative was quite high. One factor contributing to this success may be the relative ease with which caregiv-

Figure 3.10
Engagement Rate by Pathway

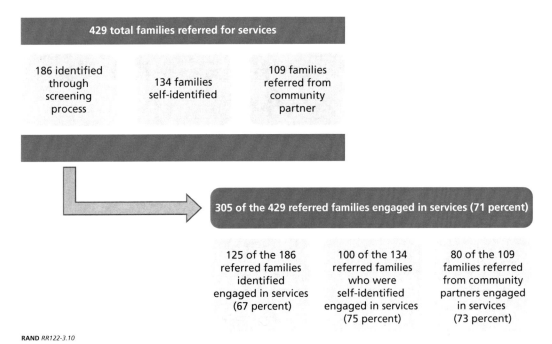

RAND RR122-3.10

ers could engage in services (e.g., in-home mobile therapy). Other factors include the "warm transfer" process, in which service coordinators or the mental health specialists directly connected caregivers to behavioral health providers, the relationship-based approach that helped caregivers understand that engaging in services for themselves would also help their child, and having the referral and connection to services coming from their service coordinator who had become a trusted resource to the family.

Engagement Types

The engagement rate varied by referral type (Figure 3.11). Most of the families referred for relationship-based services through the Part C early intervention system engaged in those services, 93 percent. Families referred to relationship-based services through the behavioral health system had engagement rates of 71 percent for team-delivered, in-home behavioral health services and 52 percent for in-home mobile therapy. Engagement rates were somewhat lower for referrals to crisis intervention (33 percent), community-based services (26 percent), and outpatient therapy (17 percent). The lower engagement rates for these referrals may partially be a result of the difficulty in obtaining follow-up information about these referrals. The Alliance was not as closely connected to the providers of those services and thus unable to readily determine engagement.

Engagement Among Caregivers with Medical Assistance

For referred caregivers on Medical Assistance, Community Care tracked data on claims for services provided by behavioral health providers in its network from March 2010 through August 2012. These data provide another perspective on engagement for a subset of the population served by the initiative and described in the preceding section. A total of 288 of the 695 caregivers who were identified for referrals were receiving Medical Assistance and were eligible to receive behavioral health services through Community Care. Of these caregivers, 210 (73 percent) had

Figure 3.11
Referrals and Engagement Rate by Type of Service

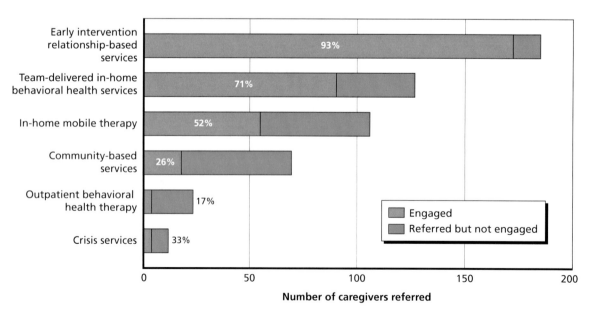

claims for services within the Community Care system. These caregivers were identified as at-risk for depression through one of the three pathways into the referral component of the initiative (Table 3.5). Forty-four percent of the caregivers with Community Care claims were identified through The Alliance depression screening process. Twenty-two percent of these caregivers self-identified a need for behavioral health or other services and supports after screening negative or declining the depression screen. The remaining 34 percent of the caregivers with Community Care claims were referred to The Alliance from community-based partners.

The caregivers on Medical Assistance with Community Care claims had their primary and secondary diagnoses documented in the Community Care system (Table 3.6). All Community Care clients who receive mental health services receive an evaluation from a provider. If the evaluation results in diagnosis, then the individual can receive treatment services. The providers are required to submit the diagnosis information to Community Care for documentation in its database, which includes comorbidities (i.e., multiple Axis I diagnoses). Sixty-one percent of caregivers had been diagnosed specifically with major depressive disorder or dysthymic disorder, and 9 percent with bipolar disorder. Caregivers also had diagnoses of anxiety disorder (22 percent), substance abuse disorder (17 percent), adjustment disorder (12 percent), and psychotic disorder (1 percent). Seven percent of caregivers had other diagnoses. Overall, 78 percent of caregivers had a diagnosis involving depression, through either a mood disorder or a component of another disorder (e.g., adjustment disorder with depressed mood.)

Of the 210 caregivers for whom claims data were available, more than one-half (n=110, 52 percent) had initiated behavioral health services before the recorded referral date suggesting that the initiative's screening and referral process did not play a role in these caregivers connecting with Community Care's behavioral health services. There were also 17 caregivers who had claims for services more than six months after the referral date. In the following analyses, we excluded both of these groups to focus on the 83 caregivers who initiated mental health services within six months of the recorded referral date because these are the caregivers who may have connected with behavioral health services because of the screening and referral process.

Table 3.5
Pathway for Caregivers with Community Care Claims

Pathway	Percentage of Caregivers (n=210)
Screening at The Alliance	44
Self-identified	22
Referral from community partner	34

Table 3.6
Diagnosis for Caregivers with Community Care Claims

Diagnosis	Percentage of Caregivers (n=210)
Major depressive disorders	61
Bipolar disorder	9
Anxiety disorder	22
Substance abuse disorder	17
Adjustment disorder	12
Psychotic disorder	1
Other disorder	7

For this group, the median time from depression screening to first mental health service was 1.4 months. It is important to note that the first paid claim date does not represent the first date of contact or service by the behavioral health provider.

The 83 caregivers with Medical Assistance who initiated services through Community Care within six months of being screened accessed a wide range of mental health and drug and alcohol services from their screening date through August 2012 (Table 3.7). More than one-half of the caregivers with Community Care claims had claims for outpatient behavioral health services (51 percent; median number of sessions=2.0) or team-delivered, in-home behavioral health services (53 percent; median number of sessions=31.5). These caregivers also had claims for medication services (27 percent; mean=5.0 sessions) which may have included pharmacologic therapy to treat depression, mobile outpatient services (39 percent; mean=5.5 sessions) and mobile crisis services (7 percent; mean=1.5 sessions). Some caregivers also had claims for inpatient mental health services (6 percent; mean=1.0 session) and service coordination (6 percent; mean=19.0 sessions) which assists adults with mental illness to develop a comprehensive recovery plan and coordinate the provision of services.

Drug and alcohol services were somewhat less common among these caregivers, with 12 percent receiving outpatient services from a drug and alcohol service provider, 4 percent receiving intensive drug and alcohol services, and 6 percent receiving methadone-related services.

Summary of the Process Measure Results

Following the initiative's screening protocol, primary caregivers of all children who received services in the Part C early intervention system were asked if they wanted to complete a depression screen. In total, 4,185 caregivers were screened for depression between February 2010 and May 2012. The overall screening rate of 63 percent of families new to The Alliance compares favorably to the depression screening rate of 53 percent for similar at-risk groups

Table 3.7
Types of Community Care Claims

Claim Type	Number of Caregivers	Percentage of Caregivers (n=83)	Range of Sessions	Median Number of Sessions/ Claims
Behavioral health services				
Outpatient services	42	51	1–95	2.0
Team-delivered in-home behavioral health services	44	53	1–85	31.5
Medication services	22	27	1–85	5.0
Mobile outpatient services	32	39	1–128	5.5
Mobile crisis services	6	7	1–5	1.5
Inpatient services	5	6	1–3	1.0
Service coordination	5	6	8–163	19.0
Drug and alcohol services				
Outpatient services	10	12	1–12	1.5
Intensive services	3	4	1–4	1.0
Methadone services	5	6	2–352	81.0
Other Services	5	6	1–2	1.0

NOTE: Number of caregivers across claim type is greater than 83 due to caregivers having multiple claim types.

(Figure 3.1; see Appendix D for full details about comparison studies). Initiative benchmarks were to screen 70 percent of caregivers during Phase 1 and 90 percent during Phase 2.

The initiative's referral component was designed to provide referrals for families identified as at risk for depression through the early intervention screening process, families who self-identified a need for support, and families who were referred to early intervention by community partners. A total of 695 families were identified for referrals through these pathways. Referrals were made for 62 percent of these families (Figure 3.12). This referral rate exceeds the average 52 percent referral rate typically among those screening positive for depression.

The initiative's engagement-in-services component focused on ensuring that caregivers who were referred for relationship-based early intervention services, behavioral health services, or other community supports received them. Overall, the engagement rate for all caregivers who received at least one referral was 71 percent, which is considerably higher than the average 37 percent engagement rate found in other studies of similar populations (Figure 3.2). Caregivers were counted as having engaged in services if the family received at least one session of one of the services for which they received a referral.

Section B. System Impact Results

To assess system impact for the second part of the evaluation, we gathered information about changes to the involved systems as a result of the implementation processes for screening and identification of at-risk families, referrals, and engagement in relationship-based services in the

Figure 3.12
Summary of Process Measure Results

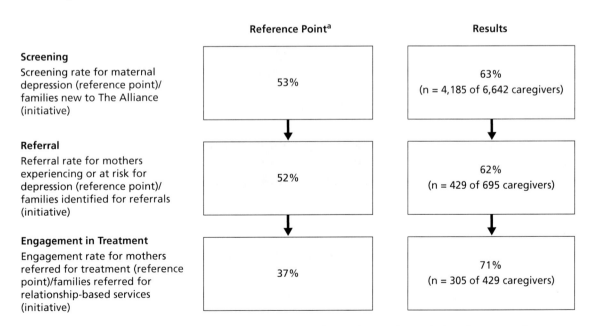

Screening
Screening rate for maternal depression (reference point)/ families new to The Alliance (initiative)

Reference Point[a]: 53%
Results: 63% (n = 4,185 of 6,642 caregivers)

Referral
Referral rate for mothers experiencing or at risk for depression (reference point)/ families identified for referrals (initiative)

Reference Point[a]: 52%
Results: 62% (n = 429 of 695 caregivers)

Engagement in Treatment
Engagement rate for mothers referred for treatment (reference point)/families referred for relationship-based services (initiative)

Reference Point[a]: 37%
Results: 71% (n = 305 of 429 caregivers)

[a] The reference points represent rates found in the literature for similar at-risk populations (e.g., screening: Armstrong and Small, 2007; Garcia, LaCaze, and Ratanasen, 2011; LaRocco-Cockburn et al., 2003; referral: Chaudron et al., 2004; Sheeder, Kabir, and Stafford, 2009; Yonkers et al., 2009; and engagement: Miranda et al., 2003; Smith et al., 2009).

Part C early intervention and behavioral health systems. The data collection involved focus groups with early intervention and behavioral health providers, telephone interviews with caregivers, and pre- and post-training surveys with initiative training participants. The system impact measures included changes in knowledge, attitudes, beliefs, and behaviors related to caregiver depression, screening, referrals, and relationship-based services, as well as perspectives from providers and caregivers on the implementation process. We synthesized the results of the system impact data collection into a series of observations on the system-level factors affecting implementation. We discuss these in detail later in this section.

Screening and Identification

Appropriate Tools and Protocols for Depression Screening. As described earlier, the depression screening tool selected for this initiative is widely used in community-based settings, easy to administer and score, and well-validated for the target population. While the screening protocol clearly articulated who should be screened, when screening should occur, and how results should be communicated, service coordinators felt that its flexibility allowed them to make adjustments depending on the particular situation or family. Nonetheless, there were challenges to completing the depression screening during early intervention home visits because of limited time or the presence of other service providers. While most caregivers felt comfortable talking about issues and stressors, some felt that service coordinators needed to spend more time building rapport and showing interest, rather than appearing to simply move through a checklist of items during the visit. Nonetheless, the consistent screening rate throughout implementation indicates that service coordinators understood and followed the protocol and caregivers accepted the depression screening as a normal part of their interaction with early intervention. This suggests that with validated tools and well-defined processes, screening for parental depression can be integrated into routine care in the Part C early intervention system.

Training and Ongoing Support for Those Conducting the Screening. The initiative undertook a range of activities to provide training and support to those conducting the screening. Some service coordinators had reservations about whether they had the skills or confidence to introduce the depression screen or engage the caregiver in a discussion about the results. To address these concerns, the training materials and sessions included specific language on introducing the screen and discussing the results, and provided the opportunity for participants to role-play different situations. In response to another concern, the local crisis services provider conducted small group meetings with service coordinators to familiarize them with services and how to access them. These training sessions helped service coordinators develop communication skills and comfort with the screening process, which eased concerns about how to effectively engage with parents on difficult topics.

Service coordinators also reported that the ongoing support from the project-funded mental health specialists provided needed consultation on the screening process, discussion of the results, and information on the local resources available to support families. Service coordinators found that as relationships developed, caregivers disclosed histories of violence and trauma. Early intervention supervisors provided further reassurance and support for providers through reflective supervision, an approach that encourages mutual sharing, reflecting, and planning as a way to increase engagement between the supervisor and service coordinator, help the provider process the experience of working with families, and partner on ways to move forward. These experiences indicate that equipping service coordinators and their supervisors with knowledge, tools, resources, and confidence in their ability to support caregivers is important for successful integration of depression screening protocols into existing processes.

Efforts to Involve the Maternal and Child Health Care System. To engage the maternal and child health care system in making referrals to early intervention based on the caregiver's depression risk, the initiative conducted outreach activities with that system to describe the initiative, establish relationships with agencies and organizations, and explain the referral process. These recruitment efforts were designed to inform providers that the Part C early intervention system was a new access point for behavioral health services for families experiencing or at risk for depression or other behavioral health issues and to describe the referral process. The results suggest that community-based child and maternal health organizations can take advantage of the system's increased capacity for screening, referral, and treatment services for caregiver depression without the volume of additional referrals exceeding the early intervention system's capacity to serve families.

Cross-System Networking and Referrals

Cross-System Networks and Communication Channels. Our current systems have evolved in a manner that fosters specialization and fragmentation in treatment and interventions. This fragmentation can result in families enlisting the help of a variety of practitioners in a serial fashion, presenting their child's same problems yet hearing interpretations through different professional lenses, inadvertently culminating in a confusing, distressing, and disheartening scenario (Lillas and Turnbull, 2009). To improve communication between systems along with referral and engagement of caregivers in services, the initiative facilitated cross-system training and networking meetings that brought together a broad group of system leaders, administrative leadership, and direct care staff to lay the groundwork for building relationships among the early intervention, behavioral health, and maternal and child health care systems. According to participants, these activities provided service providers from different systems with opportunities for face-to-face introductions and interactions where they could discuss better outcomes for the parent and young child. The development of a shared vision of system transformation among system leaders was seen as an important first step toward effective cross-system collaboration and integration. Some of these relationships had developed during the prior phase of the Collaborative's work to engage and educate the maternal and child health care system on addressing maternal depression. This initiative provided new availability of the Part C early intervention system as an access point for services and treatment for caregivers experiencing or at risk for depression.

The relationships at every level within and across systems that developed and strengthened through cross-system networking meetings were also viewed as helping administrators and providers understand the role of each system and how to support each other in providing services for at-risk families. Overall, the efforts to develop cross-system networks and communication channels increased service capacity, communication, and coordination within and between the Part C early intervention and behavioral health systems.

Integration of Referral Processes into Routine Practice. Service coordinators and supervisors found that collaborative development of a simple and clear referral process helped address the challenges in making changes to existing processes—such as resistance to new procedures, perceptions about potential increases in burden, and workload—and concerns about follow-through on referrals. In addition to the referral process, the project team developed a resource and referral guide to support the service coordinators in making referrals. While service coordinators were knowledgeable about resources that addressed early childhood developmental delays, they were often less familiar with behavioral health services for caregivers experiencing depression and with other community supports that may help both the parent and the young child. According to service coordinators, the defined referral protocols and concrete guidance about the referral options enabled knowledgeable and personalized referrals that matched needs and contributed to a high rate of referral acceptance by families.

"Warm Transfer" Process for Referrals. For those referrals to behavioral health services, the referral protocol emphasized directly connecting caregivers to these services during the early intervention home visit. This "warm transfer" strategy capitalized on the developing relationship and trust between the service coordinator and the caregiver. When the service coordinator was either able to call the provider agency with the caregiver during a visit or tell the caregiver that a specific person from the provider agency would be calling to follow up, this more direct hand-off enhanced the caregivers' comfort level with the referral process and the agency to which they were being referred. This type of referral and direct transfer from a trusted provider (i.e., an early intervention service coordinator who comes to the home) to other services and supports can increase engagement in treatment services (i.e., behavioral health providers).

Coordination and Supports for Referrals. Historically, early intervention programs focused primarily on the child's developmental delays or disabilities in terms of cognition, communication, movement, vision, and hearing. Although social/emotional development has always been an eligible domain for evaluation and treatment in early intervention, needs in this area were generally perceived as the purview of the mental health system. To increase communication and coordination of services across systems, the initiative funded two full-time mental health specialists at The Alliance. These specialists were seen as bridging the gap between early intervention, which had not previously addressed caregiver depression, and the behavioral health system. The mental health specialists provided ongoing support to strengthen relationships between providers in the Part C early intervention and behavioral health systems. Service coordinators who identified a caregiver in need of support were able to utilize a mental health specialist to identify an appropriate service or provider. The mental health specialists were also available to make providers aware of the new referrals and to give families the name of the provider who would be contacting them. The mental health specialists also offered service providers ongoing support and mentoring on the screening and referral processes. Most caregivers found the referral process to be quick and easy and felt that the service coordinator provided the support and encouragement needed to accept and follow through with the referral. However, caregivers also noted a need for improved communication and follow-up after the initial referral. Overall, providers felt that the efforts of the mental health specialists streamlined the referral process and contributed to high referral acceptance rates.

Engagement in Services for At-Risk Families

Capacity-Building Around Relationship-Based Practices. The initiative's third component focused on providing behavioral health services to caregivers that addressed behavioral health issues as well as parenting approaches and parent-child relationships, and early intervention services that considered the parent-child relationship and its impact on child development. The differing orientations in the two systems—with early intervention providers focused on the child and behavioral health providers focused on the adult—meant that providers needed to expand how they viewed their roles and responsibilities in working with families. The relationship-based models of dyadic therapies selected for the initiative—models that help parents to interpret and respond to their infants' cues, express their own emotions, and prevent or repair damage to the parent-child relationship—met the needs of the target population and aligned with the interests of the providers to work with the parent in the context of the parent-child relationship.

Behavioral health and early intervention providers were offered initial overview training on infant mental health and relationship-based care. They were then given the opportunity to pursue training in one of the three relationship-based models. These trainees shared positive impressions of the training and the value of the relationship-based approach throughout both systems, which led several agencies to request that their entire staff receive training in the models. Overall, more than 300 early intervention and behavioral health practitioners working in partner agencies were trained on relationship-based practices. These providers showed increased knowledge about effectively engaging caregivers, infant-caregiver attachment, and relationship-based care. While the relationship-based care approach helped providers in both systems focus on the parent-child relationship in their work with the family, some caregivers noted that the providers were not always equipped to meet needs or address issues. These results suggest that expanded capacity for relationship-based practice in early intervention and behavioral health, along with the two-generational approach recommended in the Institute of Medicine report, can increase engagement in services and treatment across both systems.

Peer Support and Learning Opportunities. The learning collaborative participants from the Part C early intervention and behavioral health systems found the group sessions on relationship-based practices valuable because they offered a forum for peer support, feedback, and discussion of implementing relationship-based techniques. Through this regular professional peer contact and support, the learning collaborative strengthened individual providers' skill development, knowledge, and comfort level with relationship-based care and allowed for continued interaction and relationship-building with providers from other systems.

Addressing Barriers to Treatment. The initiative also addressed some of the barriers to engagement in behavioral health treatment. Cultural context and stigma were factors considered when developing the processes for offering depression screening within early intervention and making cross-system referrals for behavioral health services and treatment. Each individual's cultural framework can affect communication about life stressors and openness to talking about issues and accessing resources and services. The screening process training sessions incorporated discussion and role playing about how to affirm caregivers' feelings, validate their distress, and offer support. The cross-system training sessions and learning collaborative activities emphasized the need to be sensitive to cultural beliefs and concerns when making referrals and supporting engagement in services and treatment.

Providing in-home behavioral health services to families in need helped address some of the typical barriers to engaging in treatment, such as lack of transportation, difficulty obtaining child care, the stigma associated with going to a clinic for mental health treatment, and the barrier of depression itself, which can make it difficult to attend traditional outpatient treatment. Community Care and the behavioral health network of providers collaborated to plan an expansion of services that would increase access to and engagement in behavioral health services for this target population. While in-home services require substantially more resources than clinic-based services, Community Care has committed to sustaining in-home service options moving forward. Overall, access to home-based behavioral health services can increase engagement rates and eliminate a significant barrier to accessing behavioral health services.

Tracking Implementation Progress and Costs

As part of the evaluation of the initiative, the project team established process measures for tracking improvements over time in depression screening, referrals, and engagement in services and treatment. This process involved The Alliance, behavioral health providers, and Community Care. The Alliance maintained a database that was shared with RAND at regular intervals for analysis and reporting. The interim results and lessons learned were discussed at periodic all-partners and funders meetings and among specific stakeholder groups. The information from these discussions was used to revise the initiative protocols.

Performance Monitoring. As with any complex initiative, it is important to incorporate ongoing assessment and monitoring of implementation in a systematic way to assess implementation progress. The regular schedule for examining the process measures (including screening, referral, and engagement in treatment or services) allowed the project team to step back and review progress on the implementation process. By continuously monitoring the implementation of the primary service delivery components, the project team identified deficiencies and worked together to develop strategies to address them. For example, screening rates did not meet expectations throughout implementation. This prompted discussions with those conducting the screening about barriers to completing the depression screening, the need for refresher training sessions, and allowing flexibility in the screening protocol.

Ongoing Quality Improvement. The project team undertook a number of activities to support ongoing quality improvement within and across systems throughout implementation. For example, after noticing that the follow-up screening rates were quite low, the data manager at The Alliance began to produce reports listing follow-up screens that were due that month and whether the families in question had been discharged from early intervention services. The supervisors and service coordinators found this information very useful in planning their visits. Since data collection for the evaluation ended, The Alliance has continued to monitor screening, referral, and engagement rates. In another effort to enable ongoing quality improvement, RAND team members led focus groups with early intervention and behavioral health providers to hear their views and suggestions on implementation of the initiative. A common issue that all providers raised in focus groups was the challenge of ongoing communication between behavioral health providers, early intervention providers, and The Alliance service coordinators. Alliance service coordinators also raised issues on the screening protocol and provided suggestions for further training and reinforcement for service coordinators. The project team used the findings from all of the focus groups to develop strategies to address the collaboration, communication, and process issues raised by those implementing the key initiative components.

Costs of Implementation. The early intervention system does incur some costs that should be considered when implementing procedures to support parental depression screening, referral, and engagement in services for families with parental depression and early childhood developmental delays. These include the cost of the depression screening tool, additional time to administer and score the screen, and the hours for training service coordinators on the screening process. Many tools for screening depression are available at no cost. Administration and scoring of the screening take only a short amount of time when incorporated into a regularly scheduled visit, and are incorporated into the family assessment component of the early intervention visit. When a parent screens positive for depression risk, service coordinators can expect to spend, on average, an extra half-hour during the visit discussing the results with the family and exploring referral options. The additional time spent linking the family to supports is a billable service coordination activity. The cost of training service coordinators to administer and score the screening tool depended on the number of staff involved and the amount of training hours conducted.

There are also early intervention system costs associated with including caregiver depression screening as a qualifying risk factor for at-risk tracking services in early intervention. The indirect costs include the time needed to train community partners in the maternal and child health care system on the referral process to early intervention. The billable costs within early intervention include those associated with the time initially required to meet with a family new to early intervention and the time associated with providing at-risk tracking services over time.

Finally, there are costs associated with cross-system networking and training activities related to conducting screening, making referrals, and providing relationship-based care. The total training costs reflect the number and type of training sessions needed to implement the different components of the initiative, including trainings on the screening and referral processes, orientation sessions for early intervention and behavioral health providers, cross-system networking meetings, relationship-based care workshops, and learning collaborative meetings. Overall, the initiative's implementation of parental depression screening in the Part C early intervention system resulted in few direct and indirect costs to The Alliance.

Family Involvement in Implementation Planning and Monitoring. The initiative's FAC provided valuable feedback throughout the planning and implementation phases to ensure the appropriateness and relevance of the initiative training materials and the informational materials on depression (e.g., an information booklet with self-help tips for caregivers), inform the development of the screening protocol and referral process, provide feedback for evaluation-related data collection (e.g., the discussion guide for the family interviews), and include a family perspective at cross-system training sessions.

In an effort to obtain feedback and suggestions from those served by The Alliance, RAND also conducted telephone interviews with caregivers who had a range of experiences related to the initiative. The interviews provided an opportunity to learn about the experiences of individual caregivers with the screening protocol, referral processes, and relationship-based services that helped in identifying strengths of the initiative and opportunities to improve implementation. Generally, caregivers identified service coordinators at The Alliance as a source of encouragement to follow through with referral and services, and they reported improved perceptions of mental health services after engaging in treatment. However, caregivers also discussed the need for improved communication with service coordinators after initial screening and referrals were in place, and for more help connecting to services beyond those coordinated by The Alliance. RAND team members communicated these findings back to the other project team members to inform improvements in the screening and referral processes.

Summary of Factors Driving System Change

The results of the system-change evaluation showed that the care system changed mainly because of three factors:

- screening and identification of families happening within early intervention
- families could access behavioral health services from the early intervention system
- early intervention and behavioral health providers were trained and supported in relationship-based care.

Section C. Individual-Level Outcome Results

The third part of the evaluation, focusing on screening and assessment, was designed to provide service coordinators with clinically useful information about depression risk and to track caregivers over time for the evaluation. In this section, we first describe the results of the baseline and follow-up depression screenings conducted. We then examine the results of the baseline and follow-up assessments that included measures of parental stress, caregiver health and safety, and child health.

Depression Screening
Baseline Depression Screening Results

Following the initiative protocol, Alliance service coordinators administered the PHQ-2 to all caregivers (n=4,185) at baseline. Those caregivers who answered "yes" to either initial screening question then completed the PHQ-9 (Figure 3.13). A total of 753 caregivers with a positive PHQ-2 completed the PHQ-9, representing 19 percent of the 4,185 caregivers screened (Figure 3.14). As shown in Figure 3.13, some caregivers completed the PHQ-9 (n=151) even though they had not responded positively to either initial screening question. In total, 904 caregivers completed the PHQ-9 at baseline.

Of the 904 caregivers with a completed PHQ-9, 44 percent screened positive (n=395) with a score of 10 or higher (representing 9 percent of the total screened). Following the initiative protocol, those who screened positive were identified for the referral component of the initiative. Studies examining positive screens in low-income mothers (e.g., Beeber et al., 2010;

Figure 3.13
Completed Baseline Screens

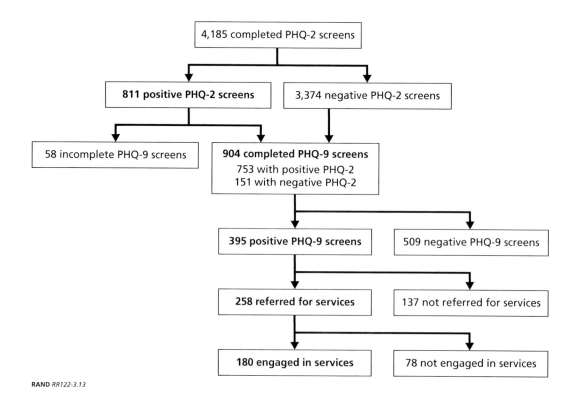

Figure 3.14
Baseline Screening Results (n=4,185)

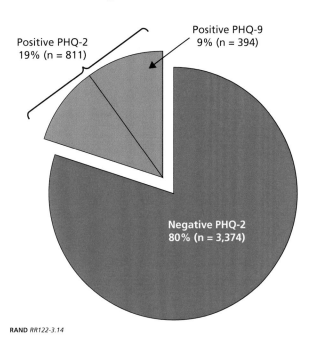

Positive PHQ-2
19% (n = 811)

Positive PHQ-9
9% (n = 394)

Negative PHQ-2
80% (n = 3,374)

Chaudron et al., 2004; Dubowitz et al., 2007; Miller, Shade, and Vasireddy, 2009; Ramos-Marcuse et al., 2010) report an average rate of 18 percent with positive screens with estimates varying across screening tools (e.g., PHQ-9, Beck Depression Inventory, Center for Epidemiologic Studies Depression Scale). Based on the literature, we expected a higher rate of positive screens than the 9 percent observed.

Among all 904 caregivers who completed the PHQ-9 at baseline, the average score (possible range 0 to 27) was 9.18 (Table 3.8). The average score among the 395 caregivers who screened positive at baseline was 15.01. According to the scoring guidelines, a score of 10–14 indicates a provisional diagnosis of minor depression while a score of 15–19 indicates a provisional diagnosis of moderately severe major depression (MacArthur Initiative for Depression and Primary Care, undated). Among the 395 who screened positive, caregivers who were referred for services (n=258) exhibited higher baseline scores than those who did not receive a referral (n=137) with means of 15.35 and 14.36, respectively. Greater referral among those with higher scores could indicate recognition of greater need by service coordinators or caregivers themselves; both played a role in determining whether a referral was ultimately made.

The analyses also explored baseline scores by whether the family had engaged in one of the relationship-based services in the Part C early intervention or behavioral health systems (Table 3.8). All families, regardless of whether they engaged in relationship-based services/ treatment, received relationship-based service coordination from The Alliance. Among caregivers who screened positive at baseline and were referred for services (n=258), baseline scores on the PHQ-9 were similar for those who engaged in relationship-based services/treatment within early intervention and/or behavioral health (n=180) and those who did not (n=78).

As noted above, not all 904 caregivers screened with the PHQ-9 at baseline received a follow-up screen. Those who did had higher scores at baseline (n=149) than those who were not screened at follow-up (n=755). This likely reflects the emphasis that the initiative placed on the

Table 3.8
Baseline PHQ-9 Scores

Group	n	Baseline Score
Caregivers completing a baseline PHQ-9 screen	904	9.18
Caregivers who screened positive	395	15.01
Caregivers who screened positive and were referred for services	258	15.35[a]
Caregivers who screened positive and were not referred for services	137	14.36[a]
Caregivers who screened positive, were referred for services and engaged in relationship-based services/treatmentb	180	15.60
Caregivers who screened positive, were referred for services but did not engage in relationship-based services/treatment[b]	78	14.78
Caregivers who completed baseline and six-month follow-up screen	149	11.39[c]
Caregivers who completed baseline, but not six-month follow-up screen	755	8.743

NOTE: Scores on the PHQ-9 range from 0 to 27.

[a] T-test indicates statistically significant difference, $t(393)=2.42$, $p<.05$.

[b] The total here is greater than 258 because some caregivers were referred for services even if they did not screen positive on the PHQ-9.

[c] T-test indicates statistically significant difference, $t(902)=-4.89$, $p<.01$.

importance of following up with caregivers who screened positive for depression. Among those caregivers who did not complete follow-up depression screens ($n=755$), 33 percent had been discharged from The Alliance prior to the date that their six-month follow-up screening was due. Taking into account those discharged before that date increases the follow-up completion rate from 16 percent to 23 percent.

The caregiver demographics were similar for those caregivers who screened at high risk for depression when compared to all caregivers who were screened (Table 3.9).

Among families in which the caregiver screened positive, the children represented similar distributions of boys and girls as well as similar age distributions (Table 3.10). However, African Americans represent a disproportionately large percentage of the caregivers who screened positive (39 percent) compared with all screened caregivers (22 percent).

Table 3.9
Caregiver Information

	Percentage of All Screens (n=4,185)	Percentage of Positive Screens (n=395)
Gender		
Female	97	98
Male	3	2
Relationship to child		
Birth parent	99	99
Adoptive parent	1	<1
Grandparent	1	<1
Other	<1	<1

NOTE: Positive screens were defined as PHQ-9 scores>10.

Table 3.10
Child Information

Characteristic	All Screens	Positive Screens
Gender	Percentage (n=4,179)	Percentage (n=391)
Female	37	38
Male	63	62
Age	Percentage (n=4,179)	Percentage (n=393)
Less than 1	42	44
1	30	29
2	28	27
Race/ethnicity	Percentage (n=3,529)	Percentage (n=355)
White (non-Hispanic)	66	45
African American (non-Hispanic)	22	39
Hispanic	2	2
Asian	3	2
Other or biracial	8	13

NOTE: Percentages do not total 100 due to rounding.

Follow-Up Depression Screening

Following the initiative protocol, Alliance service coordinators attempted to complete depression screens at baseline and at six and 12 months with rescreening conducted regardless of screening status at baseline (Table 3.11). Nearly one-third (30 percent) of the 4,185 caregivers screened at baseline also received a six-month follow-up screen with the PHQ-2. Overall, 16 percent of the 904 caregivers with baseline PHQ-9 scores completed a follow-up PHQ-9 at six months (Figure 3.15). Among the 395 caregivers who screened positive with the PHQ-9 at baseline, about one-quarter (24 percent) completed six-month follow-up depression screens. Overall, few caregivers completed 12-month follow-ups.

There are a number of explanations for the low completion rates for the follow-up depression screens. Families are discharged from the Part C early intervention system when the child reaches the age of three or when the child's functioning has improved to the point where they no longer have a developmental delay. For those discharged, The Alliance no longer had contact with the families and it was not possible to complete the follow-up screening and assessment. For some families, once connected to behavioral health services, they no longer remained involved with the at-risk tracking services offered through the Part C early intervention system, and, in turn, did not receive the follow-up screens. Service coordinators also reported that some families declined the follow-up screen because it was stressful to complete during a busy IFSP quarterly meeting or six-month review or when there were other service providers in the home.

Table 3.11
Completed Baseline and Follow-Up Depression Screens

Measure	Number Completed at Baseline	Number (Percentage) Completed at Six-Month Follow-Up	Number (Percentage) Completed at 12-Month Follow-Up
PHQ-2	4,185	1,252 (30%)	653 (16%)
PHQ-9	904	149 (50%)	88 (10%)
PHQ-9 (positive)	395	94 (24%)	55 (14%)

Figure 3.15
Completed Follow-Up Screens

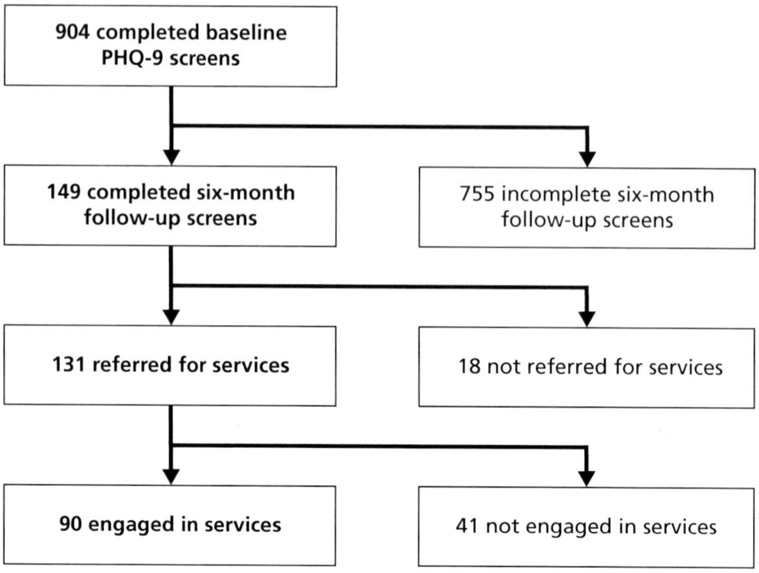

RAND *RR122-3.15*

Average PHQ-9 scores declined over time (Table 3.12). Overall, among caregivers who completed the PHQ-9 at both baseline and six months and were referred for services (n=131), scores declined by four points on the 27-point scale between baseline and the follow-up screens, with statistically significant decreases in scores from baseline to six months, baseline to 12 months, and six months to 12 months. The pattern of decreasing depressive symptoms over time held for caregivers who engaged in relationship-based services/treatment within early intervention and/or behavioral health (n=90). Among caregivers who did not engage in relationship-based services (n=41), there were statistically significant decreases in scores from baseline to six months and baseline to 12 months but not from six months to 12 months. However, the lack of difference from six to 12 months may reflect reduced statistical power. The difference in the change from baseline to six months for the two groups is discussed in more detail later. According to the scoring guidelines, a decrease of two to four points from baseline after at least three sessions of psychological counseling over four to six weeks is considered "probably inadequate" (MacArthur Initiative on Depression and Primary Care, undated). A decrease of five points from baseline is considered adequate. It is important to note that the treatment responses referenced in the PHQ-9 scoring guidelines are based on three sessions of psychological counseling. The caregivers in our analyses were counted as having engaged if they received one or more session of one of the early intervention, behavioral health, or community-based services to which they were referred.

We also conducted repeated analysis of variance measures to test for change in PHQ-9 scores across time for caregivers who received referrals and engaged in any service, as well as caregivers who received referrals but did not engage in services. For caregivers who received referrals and engaged in any service, PHQ-9 scores decreased across time (omnibus F test, $p<.01$), with change in symptoms occurring between baseline and the six-month screening ($p<.01$). PHQ-9 scores did not change significantly between the six-month screening and

Table 3.12
Changes in PHQ-9 Scores Over Time

Comparison	Caregivers Who Completed PHQ-9 at Both Time Points	Baseline Score	Six-Month Score	12-Month Score	Significance Level (t-test)
Caregivers who completed PHQ-9 at both times and were referred for services					
Baseline to six-month	131	12.37	8.37	—	p<.01
Baseline to 12-month	79	12.81	—	8.70	p<.01
Six-month to 12-month	59	—	9.75	8.24	p<.05
Caregivers who completed PHQ-9 at both times, were referred for services, and who engaged in relationship-based services/treatment					
Baseline to six-month	90	12.60	9.09	—	p<.01
Baseline to 12-month	54	13.26	—	9.31	p<.01
Six-month to 12-month	39	—	10.69	8.74	p<.05
Caregivers who completed PHQ-9 at both times, were referred for services, and who did not engage in relationship-based services/treatment					
Baseline to six-month	41	11.85	6.80	—	p<.01
Baseline to 12-month	25	11.84	—	7.36	p<.01
Six-month to 12-month	20	—	7.90	7.25	n.s.

NOTE: Scores on the PHQ-9 range from 0 to 27, significance levels indicate differences examined with a paired t-test. n.s.= non-significant.

12-month screening, suggesting that symptoms began to level off over time. There were too few caregivers who received referrals but did not engage in services to perform hypothesis testing.

As noted above, among caregivers who completed the PHQ-9 at baseline and six months, caregivers who engaged in relationship-based treatment/services (n=90) and those who did not (n=41) showed significant declines in depressive symptoms over time (Figure 3.16). This overall downward trend in depressive symptoms for both groups may reflect a general process of adjustment to the stressful situation of identifying a developmental delay for the caregiver's child, reduced parenting stress as children mature (especially for parents of very young infants), or regression to the mean. The black line shows the cut score of ten used to determine depression risk. Both groups were above the cut score at baseline but the average score for both groups decreased to below the cut score at six months. We also conducted a multiple regression analysis examining the impact of an initial PHQ-9 score, engagement status, and the interaction of these two characteristics on the PHQ-9 score at six months (see Figure 3.16). This analysis indicated that the decline in depression scores was more pronounced for those who did not engage in services than those who did. Initial PHQ-9 score and engagement status were not significant predictors of PHQ-9 score at six months when the interaction was entered into the equation (standardized beta for interaction=.80, p<.05, standardized beta for initial PHQ-9=−.05, p>.05 standardized beta for engagement status=−.44, p>.05; overall R-squared=.27). Because participant engagement in services was not randomly assigned, it may be the case that those who engage in services recognize that their needs are likely to be pervasive over the longer term. Thus, differences that appear to be due to engagement in services may be due to self-selection of participants into the engaged and not-engaged groups.

Figure 3.16
Change in PHQ-9 Scores from Baseline to Follow-Up by Engagement

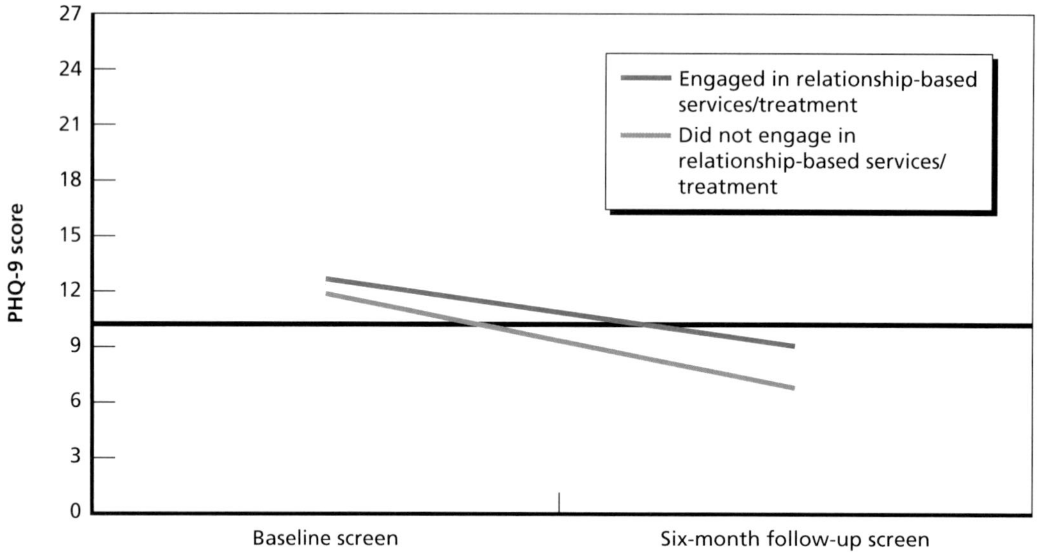

RAND *RR122-3.16*

Parenting Stress

The assessment was designed to help identify the kinds of stressors affecting the caregiver and family and the areas with the greatest need for assistance. Those caregivers screening at high risk for depression were asked to complete the PSI-SF, an assessment that contained a measure of parental stress, in addition to some caregiver health and safety items and child health items.

Baseline Parenting Stress

At baseline, these assessments were completed with a total of 401 caregivers, including 290 of the 395 caregivers who screened positive on the PHQ-9 and 111 who screened negative or did not complete the PHQ-9 (Figure 3.17).

Overall, 60 percent of the 290 caregivers who screened positive on the PHQ-9 and completed an assessment had total stress levels that fell in the clinical range, representing very high levels of stress (Figure 3.18). For the different subscales, 79 percent of the sample reached clinical levels on the parental distress subscale, 37 percent reached clinical levels on the parent-child dysfunctional interaction subscale, and 45 percent reached clinical levels on the difficult child subscale.

Among the 401 caregivers who completed the PSI-SF at baseline (possible range 36 to 180), the average score was 88.46 (Table 3.13). There were not any differences at baseline in the levels of parenting stress depending on whether a referral had been made or the family engaged in relationship-based services/treatment. There were statistically significant differences depending on whether a follow-up assessment was completed, with those receiving a follow-up assessment (n=81) having higher PSI-SF scores at baseline compared to those who did not (n=320).

Follow-Up Parenting Stress

Among the 401 caregivers who completed baseline assessments, 82 caregivers (20 percent) completed six-month follow-up assessments (Figure 3.19).

Figure 3.17
Completed Baseline Assessments

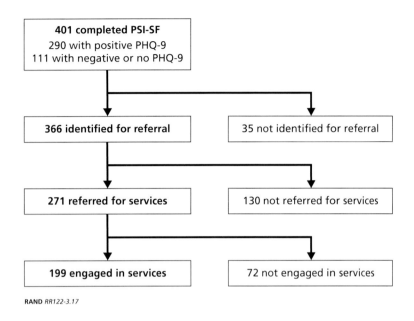

RAND *RR122-3.17*

Figure 3.18
Scores on the Parenting Stress Index Short Form (n=290)

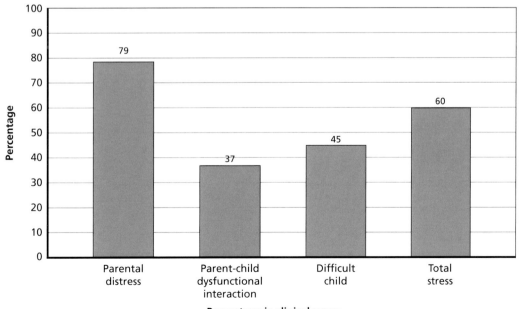

RAND *RR122-3.18*

Table 3.13
Baseline PSI-SF Scores

Group	n	Baseline Score
Caregivers completing a baseline PSI-SF	401	88.46
Caregivers completing a baseline PSI-SF who were identified as needing a referral	366	89.99
Caregivers completing a baseline PSI-SF who were referred for services	271	90.51
Caregivers completing a baseline PSI-SF who were not referred for services	95	88.48
Caregivers who completed baseline PSI-SF, were referred for services, and engaged in relationship-based services/treatment	199	91.30
Caregivers who completed a baseline PSI-SF, were referred for services, but did not engage in relationship-based services/treatment	72	88.26
Caregivers who completed baseline and six-month follow-up PSI-SF	81	83.72[a]
Caregivers who completed baseline, but not six-month follow-up PSI-SF	320	89.521

NOTE: Possible scores on the PSI-SF range from 36 to 180.

[a] T-test indicates statistically significant difference, t (399)=2.15, p<.05.

Overall, average PSI-SF scores decreased among caregivers who completed both baseline and follow-up assessments (Table 3.14). Scores declined significantly from baseline to six months and baseline to 12 months both overall and for caregivers who engaged in relationship-based services/treatment in early intervention and/or behavioral health. There were too few caregivers who did not engage in relationship-based services/treatment to perform hypothesis testing.

Health and Safety

Caregivers who screen at high risk for depression also answered a series of questions about their health and safety and their children's health. Forty-one percent of these caregivers rated their overall health status as "fair" or "poor" (Figure 3.20). In comparison, a 2008 study of Penn-

Figure 3.19
Completed Follow-Up Assessments

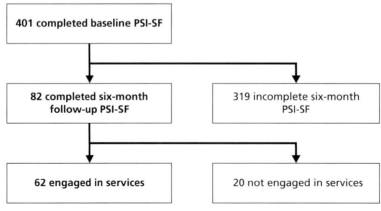

RAND RR122-3.19

Table 3.14
Change in PSI-SF Scores Over Time

Comparison	Caregivers Who Completed PSI-SF at Both Time Points	Baseline Score	Six-Month Score	12-Month Score	Significance Level (t-test)
Caregivers who completed PSI-SF at both times					
Baseline to six-month	82	83.52	77.33		p<.01
Baseline to 12-month	55	89.25		82.53	p<.01
Six-month to 12-month	48		78.44	77.92	n.s.
Caregivers who completed PSI-SF at both times who engaged in relationship-based services/treatment					
Baseline to six-month	62	85.53	78.10		p<.01
Baseline to 12-month	39	92.31		85.97	p<.05
Six-month to 12-month	34		78.53	80.26	n.s.

NOTE: n.s.=non-significant.

sylvania adults found that 16 percent considered themselves to be in "fair" or "poor" health (Bureau of Health Statistics and Research, 2009).

On the assessment, caregivers who screened at high risk for depression were also asked about the number of days in the last month in which they had inadequate rest or sleep (Figure 3.21). The vast majority of these caregivers (91 percent) indicated that they did not get adequate sleep more than seven days in the past month, including 83 percent who had inadequate sleep for 15 or more days. In comparison, a recent study with a similar population that used a threshold for "inadequate" sleep of 14 or more days in the past month found that 36 percent of unmarried mothers, 34 percent of married mothers, and 39 percent of women with three or more children reported insufficient sleep (Chapman et al., 2012).

Figure 3.20
Caregiver Overall Health (n=302)

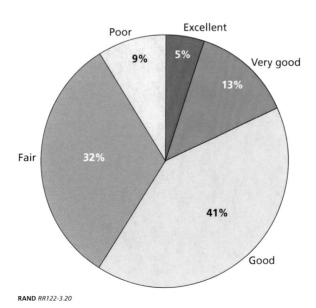

RAND RR122-3.20

Figure 3.21
Caregiver Number of Days Without Adequate Sleep in the Last 30 Days (n=290)

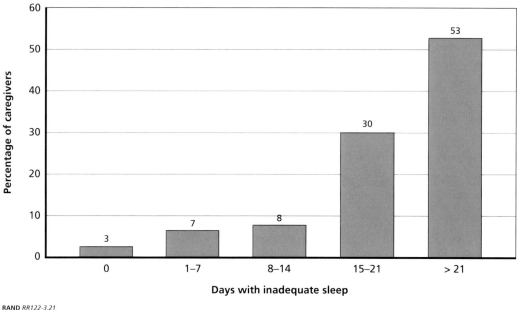

RAND *RR122-3.21*

Caregivers who screened at high risk for depression reported poor diets compared with the overall U.S. adult population. Only 8 percent of these caregivers reported a "very good" or "excellent" diet (Figure 3.22). This compares to 33 percent of Americans reporting a "very good" or "excellent" diet in 2006 (U.S. Department of Agriculture, 2009).

Figure 3.22
Caregiver Overall Diet (n=303)

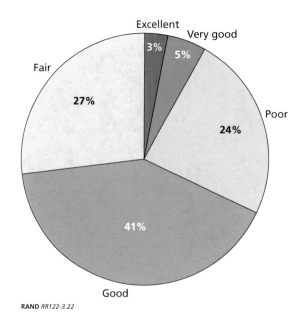

RAND *RR122-3.22*

Nearly half of those who screened at high risk for depression (46 percent) had not engaged in physical activity during the past month. This compares with 26 percent of Pennsylvania adults who indicated that they had not engaged in any leisure time physical activity in the past month (Bureau of Health Statistics and Research, 2009).

The vast majority of caregivers who screened positive had access to routine or preventive health care (Figure 3.23). More than half (53 percent) went to a doctor's office or accessed care through their health maintenance organization while 24 percent went to a clinic or health center for routine health care. Overall, 23 percent of the caregivers did not have a usual place of health care. This is comparable to national statistics that show 17 percent of U.S. adults do not have a usual place of health care. Nationally, of those with a usual place of care, three-quarters received care at a doctor's office or health maintenance organization, 21 percent went to a clinic or health center, and 3 percent used a hospital emergency room or outpatient department for routine or preventive health care (Pleis, Ward, and Lucas, 2010).

Among families with a caregiver who screened positive for depression, about one-half of caregivers (53 percent) and children (47 percent) had one or more emergency room visits during the prior six months (Figure 3.24). In comparison, nationally in 2007, 20 percent of adults aged 18 and over had one or more emergency room visits (National Center for Health Statistics, 2009). For children under the age of four, 73 percent had no visits, 18 percent had one visit, and 9 percent had two or more visits in 2009 (Bloom, Cohen, and Freeman, 2009).

In terms of routine and preventive health care for children of caregivers who screened positive for depression, 94 percent had a regular physician and 95 percent had up-to-date immunizations. Nationally, in 2008, 4 percent of U.S. children did not have a usual source of care. The estimated vaccination rate for children 19–36 months old is 90 percent or higher (Bloom, Cohen, and Freeman, 2009).

Figure 3.23
Caregiver Routine or Preventive Care (n=300)

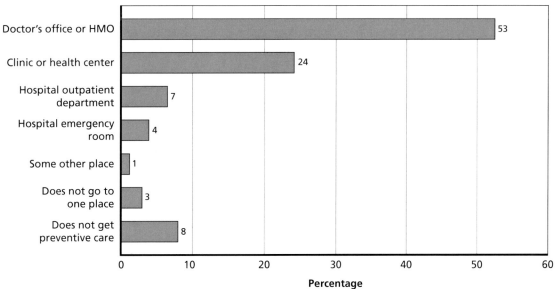

Figure 3.24
Emergency Room Visits (n=290 for caregiver, n=279 for child)

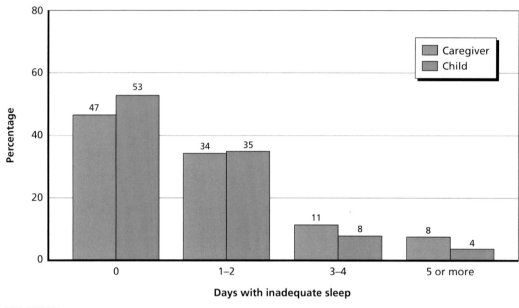

RAND RR122-3.24

The assessment also asked about the caregiver's safety. Less than 3 percent of the caregivers who screened at high risk for depression reported being in an unsafe relationship, although 10 percent of the caregivers who screened at high risk for depression reported a history of domestic violence.

The service coordinators also attempted to administer the health and safety portion of the assessment at six and 12 months. An analysis of responses at both time points indicates that caregivers perceived their physical health, diet, sleep, and access to routine health care had improved between the baseline and follow-up assessment (Table 3.15). The changes over time were not analyzed by engagement in services because of the small number of caregivers in the group who did not engage in service but completed a follow-up assessment.

Overall, those caregivers who completed these items at baseline and six months showed improvement in some of the self-reported caregiver health measures, including physical health, diet, sleep, and access to routine health care, although the sample sizes were quite small.

Summary of the Individual Outcome Measure Results

The screening and assessment component of the initiative was designed to identify caregivers with depressive symptoms and to assess their parenting stress and health situation. The baseline screening results show that 9 percent of caregivers screened positive for depression with the two-step screening protocol. Those caregivers screening at high risk for depression were administered an assessment with a measure of parental stress as well as health and safety items. Overall, 60 percent of the caregivers with positive screens who completed an assessment had total parental stress in the "clinical" range, representing very high levels of stress. These caregivers also reported inadequate sleep as well as worse perceived health, poorer diet, and less physical activity than comparison populations.

Table 3.15
Changes in Health Outcomes Over Time

Health Outcome	Baseline Score	Follow-Up Score	Significance Level
Physical health (n=88) *1 (excellent) to 5 (poor) scale*	3.14	2.91	p<.05
Diet (n=87) *1 (excellent) to 5 (poor)*	3.71	3.43	p<.01
Sleep (n=80) *Number of days without adequate sleep in the past month*	21.75	16.31	p<.01
Physical activity (n=88) *Percentage who engaged in physical activity in the past month*	51	57	n.s.
Emergency room visits—caregiver (n=82) *Number of visits in past 6 months*	1.45	0.89	n.s.
Emergency room visits—child (n=81) *Number of visits in past 6 months*	0.91	0.88	n.s.
Access to routine health care—caregiver (n=86) *Percentage who indicated that they had a regular provider*	77	87	p<.05
Access to routine health care—child (n=80) *Percentage who indicated that the child had a regular provider*	97	95	n.s.
Vaccinations (n=82) *Percentage who reported child is up to date on immunizations*	96	94	n.s.

NOTE: n.s.=non-significant.

Tracking caregivers over time proved somewhat challenging. Only 24 percent of those who screened at high risk for depression at baseline completed a follow-up screen, although some of these families had been discharged from The Alliance prior to the follow-up screening due date. Among caregivers who completed the baseline parenting stress measure, 20 percent had a follow-up assessment. In general, among caregivers for whom both baseline and six-month follow-up data were available, depressive symptoms decreased over time. This decrease was found among caregivers who completed the PHQ-9 at both times. The decline in depressive symptoms over time may reflect a general process of adjustment to the stressful situation of identifying a developmental delay for the caregiver's child.

Caregivers who ultimately engaged in relationship-based services/treatment showed higher levels of depressive symptoms at baseline than those who did not, suggesting that those with greater need may be more likely to take advantage of the services being offered through the initiative. Both those who engaged and those who did not engage showed improvement in their depressive symptoms over time. In contrast, there were not any differences at baseline in the levels of parenting stress depending on whether a referral had been made or the family engaged in services. While only caregivers who engaged in relationship-based services/treatment showed an improvement in parenting stress over time, the small sample size for those that did not engage limits the ability to detect a difference. Caregivers also showed improvement in self-reported health measures, including physical health, diet, sleep, and access to routine health care.

Despite the overall low retention rate for screening at six months, it appears that depressive symptoms decreased over time for those caregivers screened at both time points. However, both those who engaged in relationship-based services/treatment within early intervention and/or behavioral health and those who did not showed improvement in their depressive symptoms. These findings suggest that caregivers involved in the initiative experienced better outcomes at six months regardless of whether they engaged in relationship-based services other than the relationship-based service coordination within early intervention.

Summary of the Results of the Overall Initiative

Historically, early intervention programs focused primarily on the child's developmental delays or disabilities in terms of cognition, communication, movement, vision, and hearing. Although social/emotional development has always been an eligible domain for evaluation and treatment in early intervention, needs in this area were generally perceived as the purview of the mental health system. Knowledge from the field of infant mental health is transforming assessment, intervention, and collaboration; as a result, families may experience a more integrated service model where fewer calls need to be made, fewer applications need to be completed, and evaluations and assessments may be shared rather than repeated. With *Helping Families Raise Healthy Children,* the Part C early intervention system screened and identified, provided referrals, and supported engagement in services for families with caregivers at risk for or experiencing depression and children experiencing or at risk for developmental delays. The evaluation assessed the implementation by examining process measures for the three initiative components; the factors that affected implementation; the system-change process; and individual-level outcome measures of depressive symptoms, parental stress, health, and safety. While it is not possible to disentangle the relationships between the implementation strategies and the process, system impact, and individual-level outcomes achieved (see limitations section in Chapter Four), the initiative successfully implemented key components and improved key processes across systems.

Discussion

The *Helping Families Raise Healthy Children* initiative aimed at addressing the related challenges of parental depression and early childhood developmental delays. Our evaluation of the initiative focused on assessing the implementation process, examining changes in individual outcomes, and identifying certain key elements that influenced implementation and contributed to systems change. In this chapter, we describe the key lessons learned from the initiative. We also provide a brief review of the current policy context to inform the development of practice and policy recommendations to sustain this work. We conclude this chapter with some observations about the limitations of our work.

Lessons Learned

The lessons presented here reflect the results of the initiative evaluation and the quality improvement and monitoring activities. They should provide guidance for other communities seeking to implement depression screening within the Part C early intervention system, strengthen cross-system collaborations, implement relationship-based care in the early intervention and behavioral health systems, and support engagement in services and treatment. For other communities interested in these processes, an implementation toolkit provides guidance, information, and resources (Schultz et al., 2012).

Screening and Identification

- **Screening for caregiver depression using validated tools can be integrated into routine care in the Part C early intervention system.** Successful implementation of depression screening during an early intervention home visit requires balancing limited time, competing demands, and the possible presence of other service providers or family members.
- **Screening for depression and referral for services is acceptable to caregivers.** Systematic depression screening in early intervention can help to identify caregivers experiencing depression, normalize the screening process for caregivers, and streamline the process of connecting caregivers to behavioral health treatment or other care needs.
- **There are multiple pathways into referral and treatment for caregiver depression.** Discussing how the caregiver feels during the screening process opens a dialogue and offers an opportunity for caregivers who decline the screen or screen negative to self-identify a need for services and support. Further, the Part C early intervention system's

increased capacity for screening, referral, and treatment services provides a place for community-based child and maternal health organizations to refer families identified as being at risk for caregiver depression and embodies the Part C enabling legislation and models of service.

- **Expanding the scope of early intervention increases opportunities for identifying early childhood developmental delays.** The addition of caregiver depression as a qualifying risk factor for early intervention at-risk tracking services has value as a means to identify and link children to needed services.

Referrals

- **Referrals are possible when accompanied by the necessary structures and supports.** Established relationships between providers across systems, well-defined referral protocols, and open communication channels are important components to a successful referral network. Integration of the referral procedures into existing procedures promotes sustainability of system changes.
- **Cross-system networking opportunities are important for fostering a sense of connection and understanding.** Training sessions and networking meetings with providers working in different systems help to establish and maintain relationships across systems and educate providers about the procedures and approaches employed in different systems. A learning collaborative model provides regular opportunities for providers across systems to establish and strengthen valuable relationships.
- **Strong relationships and trust between providers and caregivers are key to successful referrals.** The strength of the relationship with the provider can improve caregiver acceptance of, and follow-through on, referrals following the initial screening. Referrals and warm transfers from a trusted provider to other services and supports can increase access to, and engagement in, services and treatment.

Engagement in Services for At-Risk Families

- **The barriers to accessing behavioral health services are not insurmountable.** Home-based behavioral health services can increase accessibility by alleviating issues such as transportation, child care, and the ability to initiate and follow through with outpatient treatment because of depressive symptoms.
- **Coordination among the providers working with a family is critical to maintaining engagement.** The providers working with a family need to communicate and coordinate services to ensure that the family's needs are met and that the situations do not become overwhelming for the family.
- **Expanded capacity for relationship-based practice can increase engagement in treatment services.** Providers will take advantage of opportunities to learn about relationship-based care and how to effectively engage families. Providers should focus on the parent-child relationship and the link with child development to help encourage parents in disclosing depression and/or parenting stress, and to provide motivation for engaging in services or treatment.

Education, Training, and Support

- **Implementation of depression screening in a new system requires intensive education, training, and support.** Those conducting the screening need initial education on depression and its effect on child development; initial training and ongoing support with the screening process; access to consultation and supervision; and education about local resources available to families, including crisis services, domestic violence resources, and behavioral health and community social service supports.
- **Cross-system trainings and supports are essential for introducing new training concepts across systems.** Cross-system training sessions offer opportunities to initiate interaction between early intervention and behavioral health providers and allow for providers to learn how referral procedures and approaches will be employed in different systems. Individual interactions at training sessions foster a sense of connection and understanding across systems that can facilitate referrals.

Current Policy Context

Created to enhance the development of infants and toddlers and the capacity of families to meet their children's needs, the federal Part C legislation guides early intervention services and provides a framework for an initiative such as *Helping Families Raise Healthy Children*. Although Part C specifies numerous minimum components required for early intervention services, states have discretion in setting the criteria for child eligibility. For example, Pennsylvania's requirements for early intervention (25 percent delay or clinical opinion) enable a significant portion of children who are at risk for developmental delays to receive treatment compared to other states where the child must have a delay of at least 50 percent in one or more areas. Beyond that, the development of infants/toddlers not currently eligible for intervention services can be monitored through at-risk tracking services if certain risk factors are present. These at-risk tracking services regularly monitor the child for the emergence of any developmental delays and link families to services as soon as a need is identified. In Pennsylvania, the following risk factors are currently included:

- Child's birth weight under 1,500 grams.
- Child cared for in a neonatal intensive care unit.
- Child born to a chemically dependent mother and referred by a physician, health care provider, or parent.
- Child is seriously abused or neglected, as substantiated and referred by the county children and youth agency.
- Child has confirmed dangerous levels of lead poisoning as set by the Department of Health.

Nationally, the early intervention legislation does not provide support for parental depression screening within the early intervention system. However, regulations released in 2011 encourage states to increase opportunities for children under three years of age who are at risk for developmental delays. Further, some states have recognized parental depression as an eligible risk factor for tracking early childhood development. While Pennsylvania does not currently recognize parental depression as a qualifying risk factor, its Child Find mandate specifies that in order to identify all at-risk children, counties should coordinate with other systems and efforts (e.g., preschool programs, maternal and child health programs, Head Start, county behavioral health programs).

Limitations

Community-based quality improvement initiatives are designed to solve a unique problem in a specific location or to understand what changes are required in order to solve it. By definition, the evaluation of such initiatives does not adhere to the gold standard of research because they are not conducted in carefully controlled laboratories, do not randomly assign participants to treatment or control groups, focus on a specific target population, and have goals that are specific to the unique problems of a particular setting. Because this is not a randomized control trial, we are not able to draw conclusions that any changes observed are the result of the initiative. Nonetheless, with these caveats in mind, the lessons derived from this evaluation of a community-based quality improvement initiative provide important information on external validity, implementation, and sustainability that can be used to inform solutions for similar problems in different contexts and advance broader efforts to improve overall systems performance. In designing the *Helping Families Raise Healthy Children* initiative, the project team carefully documented the implementation process and designed quality monitoring and evaluation activities with a clear set of methods and approaches that can be easily adapted and applied to other communities in Pennsylvania that undertake similar systems-change efforts, and to disseminate detailed findings regarding what was done, what was modified during implementation, what worked, and why—with the ultimate goal of informing policy and practice change at the state level.

There are several limitations to the design of the initiative that should be considered. First, there were a number of limitations associated with the evaluation's data-collection activities for the process measures. For example, we used the perinatal and postpartum depression literature to establish reference points for the initiative because empirical evidence regarding caregiver depression and its effects on child development is sparse in the early intervention field. While these reference points provided context for the initiative and established reference points for our quality improvement efforts, the populations differ (e.g., the cause of depression may differ, development is influenced during the prenatal and postpartum period). However, because the focus of the initiative was on system improvements rather than determining the cause of depression or child developmental delays, these limitations do not alter the interpretations of our findings. Relatedly, the definition of referral and engagement in the referent studies varied. For example, while most studies did not explicitly define referral, that term typically referred to the participant receiving a recommendation for a specific provider or service. Further, due to the nature of family tracking and intake into the Part C early intervention system, it was challenging to establish a reliable denominator for calculating the overall screening rate. Data collection limitations also necessitated a liberal definition of engagement in services. For each referred family, The Alliance attempted to confirm whether the family had received the service but was unable to determine the number of sessions received. As a result, engagement was defined as having received at least one session.

Second, for the system impact measures, the training evaluation was relatively narrow in scope and primarily measured change in knowledge and participant satisfaction with the training. Data on the impact of the training on provider practice behaviors would have yielded more definitive information on the effectiveness of the initiative training. Finally, we did not measure whether and how providers used the relationship-based models in their work with families. As a result, we cannot assess how the practice or quality of their delivery changed.

Third, for the individual outcome measures, the initiative was limited in its ability to determine whether screening, referral, and engagement in services were directly associated with improved individual-level outcomes. As part of the initiative, all caregivers (i.e., caregivers in the Part C early intervention system or referred from community care providers) were eligible for depression screening, and all who screened positive or who self-identified a need for support were eligible for referrals and engagement in relationship-based services. By design, the initiative lacked a true comparison group of caregivers who were not offered screening or the opportunity to be referred for services or supports. Because depression scores decreased for all caregivers (those who engaged in both relationship-based services and service coordination and those who engaged only in relationship-based service coordination), it is unclear how much the implementation of systematic depression and referral processes affect risk for depression over time. However, a design that would allow for such comparisons was contrary to the Collaborative's primary interest of improving the processes related to screening, referral, and engagement in services for all caregivers experiencing or at risk for depression. This component of the evaluation was also constrained by challenges in collecting follow-up data on caregivers screened at baseline. The completion rates for follow-up assessments were quite low for reasons that included caregiver refusal, the family's discharge from early intervention services or at-risk tracking, and inability to contact the family.

CHAPTER FIVE

Conclusions, Recommendations, and Next Steps

Moving forward, the challenge for the *Helping Families Raise Health Children* initiative will be to continue its successful components while addressing the remaining challenges. In this concluding chapter, we first describe the sustainability plans for the initiative, then provide policy and practice recommendations for different stakeholder groups to capitalize on its successful system-change efforts.

Sustainability of the Initiative's Components

Since its inception, the Allegheny County Maternal and Child Health Care Collaborative has been driven by a shared vision of transforming systems to improve the lives of families with young children in the community. For the *Helping Families Raise Healthy Children* initiative, the leadership and guidance of local and state policymakers has enabled the Collaborative to drive system change both locally and across the state. Providers and practices from the Part C early intervention and behavioral health systems have effectively collaborated to improve processes and procedures, build system capacity, and find solutions to the challenges inherent in changing how systems work and work together.

Based on the successful implementation of *Helping Families Raise Healthy Children*, the Collaborative partners plan to sustain the screening, referral, and engagement-in-service components beyond the initiative through practice and policy changes. The Allegheny County Office of Behavioral Health and the Regional Office of Child Development and Early Learning are supportive of recognizing primary caregiver depression as an eligible risk factor for early intervention at-risk tracking services. Allegheny County plans to add "caregiver depression" as an eligible risk factor for at-risk tracking services to its Annual Early Intervention plan, thus ensuring the sustainability of this important component of the initiative.

The integration of screening, referral, and services into existing structures supports the sustainability of these new processes and protocols. The Alliance will continue using the screening protocol developed for the initiative to offer depression screening to all families receiving early intervention services. The Alliance will also continue to accept referrals from community-based agencies in the maternal and child health care system for developmental assessment and services with the addition of caregiver depression as an eligible risk factor. For those families identified as needing support and services, service coordinators are being trained to provide relationship-based service coordination and referrals. The cross-system networks and communication channels established through the initiative provide a foundation for continued collaboration and coordination to ensure that families are connected to needed services. For the services component, the initiative's ability to expand capacity for mobile mental health services and relationship-based practice in both systems increased access to, and engagement in, treatment for families experiencing parental depression and early childhood developmental delays. Both systems are committed to continuing the training and education efforts around relationship-based practice. The relationship-based and mobile services and treatment within behavioral health are sustainable through Medicaid reimbursement.

Overall, the integration of new protocols into existing service structures and the establishment of cross-systems relationships strengthened the sustainability of all initiative components. Based on our on-the-ground experience implementing *Helping Families Raise Healthy Children*, the project team produced "A Toolkit for Implementing Parental Depression Screening, Referral, and Treatment Across Systems" (Schultz et al., 2012). The toolkit provides step-by-step recommendations for developing a cross-systems approach to address parental depression, including screening for depression in early intervention, developing networking and referral processes, and providing relationship-based care within the early intervention and behavioral health systems. Using the resources and materials in the toolkit, several Pennsylvania counties have begun the process of planning and implementing depression screening and referrals, as well as a relationship-based approach to services within the Part C early intervention and behavioral health systems.

Recommendations

The *Helping Families Raise Healthy Children* initiative was designed as a cross-systems effort to improve quality and change the way local systems serve families experiencing the related and often co-occurring challenges of parental depression and early childhood developmental delays. The initiative's success in screening and identifying caregiver depression, developing networking and referral processes, and providing relationship-based care within the Part C early intervention and behavioral health systems demonstrates the viability of a systems-change approach. The results of the initiative suggest policy and practice recommendations in three areas:

1. improving screening and identification of caregiver depression (Table 5.1)
2. enhancing cross-system referral and coordination (Table 5.2)
3. increasing engagement in services and treatment (Table 5.3).

These recommendations are meant to provide a framework for moving the relevant systems toward a more integrated and coordinated approach to caregiver depression and early childhood developmental delays. They are targeted toward decisionmakers and practitioners at the state, county, and provider levels, depending on the jurisdiction. For each area of policy and practice, we present recommendations for the following stakeholder groups with the relevant Pennsylvania stakeholder group named in parentheses:

- State Legislature (Pennsylvania General Assembly)
- State and/or county early intervention agencies (Pennsylvania Department of Public Welfare, Office of Child Development and Early Learning; county early intervention coordination units)

Table 5.1
Recommendations to Improve Screening and Identification of Caregiver Depression

Stakeholder	Recommendation
State legislature (Pennsylvania General Assembly)	• Mandate universal screening for depression in the Part C early intervention system. • Add parental mental health challenges as a qualifying factor for early intervention at-risk tracking services statewide.
State and/or county early intervention agencies (Pennsylvania Department of Public Welfare, Office of Child Development and Early Learning; county early intervention coordination units)	• Support referral of infants and toddlers in families with a primary caregiver at risk for depression to early intervention for developmental screening. • Add depression as tracking category for early intervention services. • Develop protocols for depression screening using a validated screening tool. • Provide initial and ongoing training and support on depression screening to service coordinators implementing the screening protocol. • Establish performance monitors to assess progress and develop strategies for improving screening rates.
State and/or county behavioral health agencies (Pennsylvania Department of Public Welfare, Office of Mental Health and Substance Abuse Services; county behavioral health administrators	• Support referral of infants and toddlers in families with a primary caregiver experiencing or at risk for depression to early intervention for developmental screening.
Behavioral health provider agencies	• Refer infants and toddlers in families with a primary caregiver experiencing or at risk for depression to early intervention for developmental screening. • Provide initial and ongoing training and support on caregiver depression, its effect on child development, and the need for developmental screening and assessment for the child.
Providers within the maternal and child health care system	• Provide depression screening using a validated tool. • Refer infants and toddlers in families with a primary caregiver at risk for depression to early intervention for developmental screening.

- Early intervention provider agencies
- State and/or county behavioral health agencies (Pennsylvania Department of Public Welfare, Office of Mental Health and Substance Abuse Services; county behavioral health administrators)
- Behavioral health provider agencies
- Physical health managed care organizations
- Providers within the maternal and child health care system.

Next Steps

The *Helping Families Raise Healthy Children* initiative represents the fourth phase of the Allegheny County Maternal and Child Health Care Collaborative's efforts to change and integrate systems for parents and children in the community. While the planned integration and sustainability of the screening and identification, referral, and engagement-in-services components are notable, the work is not completed. The Collaborative is committed to continuing its efforts to transform systems within Allegheny County and to serving as a catalyst for other communities across the Commonwealth of Pennsylvania.

Table 5.2
Recommendations to Enhance Cross-System Referral and Coordination

Stakeholder	Recommendation
State and/or county early intervention agencies (Pennsylvania Department of Public Welfare, Office of Child Development and Early Learning; county early intervention coordination units)	• Promote cross-system collaboration and communication among the early intervention, behavioral health, and maternal and child health care systems. • Develop cross-system referral protocols for families identified as needing behavioral health services and other supports. • Facilitate cross-system collaboration and communication among providers in the early intervention, behavioral health, and maternal and child health care systems. • Provide initial training and ongoing support to service coordinators on cross-system referral protocols. Establish performance monitors to assess progress and develop strategies for improving the cross-system referral process.
Early intervention provider agencies	• Facilitate networking and communication with providers in the behavioral health and maternal and child health care systems.
State and/or county behavioral health agencies (Pennsylvania Department of Public Welfare, Office of Mental Health and Substance Abuse Services; county behavioral health administrators)	• Promote cross-system collaboration and communication among the early intervention, behavioral health, and maternal and child health care systems. • Develop cross-system referral protocols for families identified as needing behavioral health services and other supports. • Facilitate cross-system collaboration and communication among providers in the early intervention, behavioral health, and maternal and child health care systems.
Behavioral health provider agencies	• Facilitate networking and communication with providers in the early intervention and maternal and child health care systems.
Behavioral health managed care organizations	• Support cross-system collaboration and communication among the early intervention, behavioral health, and maternal and child health care systems.

Table 5.3
Recommendations to Increase Engagement in Services and Treatment

Stakeholder	Recommendation
State and/or county early intervention agency (Pennsylvania Department of Public Welfare, Office of Child Development and Early Learning; county early intervention coordination units)	• With behavioral health, implement a training curriculum for providers from both systems on the interconnectedness of caregiver depression and early childhood developmental delays, the science of early childhood brain development, the impact of toxic stress, relationship-based care practices, and reflective supervision.
Early intervention provider agencies	• Provide ongoing support and reflective supervision for providers on relationship-based approaches to working with families.
State and/or county behavioral health agencies (Pennsylvania Department of Public Welfare, Office of Mental Health and Substance Abuse Services; county behavioral health administrators	• With early intervention, implement a training curriculum for providers from both systems on the interconnectedness of caregiver depression and early childhood developmental delays, the science of early childhood brain development, the impact of toxic stress, and relationship-based care practices. • Support expansion of in-home behavioral health services for families with caregivers at risk for or experiencing depression and infants/toddlers at risk for developmental delays.
Behavioral health provider agencies	• Expand capacity to provide in-home behavioral health services. • Provide initial and ongoing training and education for providers on relationship-based approaches to working with families.
Behavioral health managed care organizations	• Allow access to in-home behavioral health services for families with caregivers at risk for or experiencing depression and infants/toddlers at risk for developmental delays.

Training Assessments

At the system level, the *Helping Families Raise Healthy Children* initiative's cross-system training efforts were designed to integrate and coordinate efforts to serve families with caregivers at risk for or experiencing depression and children at risk for developmental delays. Training was available to local maternal and child health care, early intervention, and behavioral health providers, and each session addressed one or more topics related to achieving the initiative's objectives (e.g., caregiver screening/assessment, referrals, relationship-based interventions) along with the importance of conducting these activities in a manner that honors and respects family values and priorities, and builds trusting relationships with families.

Training Session Overview

The early initiative trainings focused on training Alliance service coordinators and supervisors on the screening/assessment process and the referral process. Table A.1 below details the training topics, number and type of participants, and the survey response rates for each training topic. Survey response rates were 100 percent for the screening/assessment process training and 84 percent for the referral process training. Additionally, follow-up training on the screening/assessment/referral process was provided to 60 service coordinators over two sessions.

More than 200 participants—made up of service coordinators and supervisors from The Alliance, behavioral health providers, and early intervention providers—attended the overview on relationship-based interventions. The lower survey response rate of 51 percent for the overview training survey may be related to the fact that this session was conducted as a single, large, training session that lasted much of the workday. In contrast, the topic-specific training sessions conducted for each of the three relationship-based intervention models that followed (Nurturing Parent, Promoting First Relationships, and Partners in Parenting Education) were shorter and utilized smaller groups.

After the initial training sessions for each of the three relationship-based interventions, additional training was provided in response to demand from individual service providers and groups. The project team provided five additional sessions on the Promoting First Relationships model of relationship-based care for 120 early intervention providers and Alliance service coordinators. The early intervention providers were interested in and enthusiastic about this particular intervention model because of its flexible approach, which offers a philosophy for relationship-based care, rather than a structured curriculum. Response rates for surveys on the three relationship-based interventions ranged from more than 90 percent for the trainings in Promoting First Relationships and Partners in Parenting Education, to

Table A.1
Initiative Trainings

Training Dates	Topic	Trainees	Number of Participants	Survey Response Rate (percentage)
November 17 and 19, 2009	Screening/Assessment Tools	Alliance service coordinators and supervisors	58	100
February 16, 19, and 23, 2010.	Referral Processes	Alliance service coordinators and supervisors	51	84
April 12, 2010	Overview of Relationship-Based Interventions	Alliance service coordinators and supervisors, behavioral health providers, early intervention providers	211	51
June 17 and 18, 2010	Nurturing Parenting	Behavioral health providers, early intervention providers	19	37
July 12 and 13, 2010, September 27, 2010, June 7, 10, and 24, 2011	Promoting First Relationships	Behavioral health providers, early intervention providers	157	97
September 14, 2010	Partners in Parenting Education	Behavioral health providers, early intervention providers	27	93

around 37 percent for the Nurturing Parent training. The lower response rate for the Nurturing Parenting training was attributed to logistical challenges to administering the survey at this particular training.

An important determinant of the success of this initiative was the adequacy of training to support the primary objectives of (1) improving the screening and identification of caregivers at risk for or experiencing depression; (2) enhancing access to support and services for these families by establishing a referral process; and (3) better serving these families by offering integrated, relationship-based treatment options that address the needs of both caregivers and young children in the context of the parent-child relationship. Data collection for the impact measures focused on pre- and post-training surveys at each initiative training session to assess knowledge, attitudes, beliefs, and behaviors (i.e., screening, referral, and engagement in treatment) related to relationship-based care. For all trainings, surveys were administered before the training session began and immediately following its completion. To evaluate training efforts, we examined differences in pre- and post-training surveys, which measured participants' knowledge, confidence in implementing skills or techniques relevant to the training, comfort in performing tasks relevant to the training—and, in some cases, attitudes toward evidence-based practices—all of which were expected to change because of the training. Participant information, such as area of expertise, was collected in the pre-training survey. These evaluations establish the impact of the training sessions, describe the characteristics of the individuals who attended the trainings, and identify areas for future improvement.

Detailed below are the training evaluation results for screening and assessment training, referral training, the overview training on infant mental health and relationship-based interventions, and each of the three relationship-based interventions. Participant characteristics and descriptive information about survey responses are provided in each section. When warranted, paired t-tests were conducted to test for pre-and post-training differences. We limited these comparisons to trainings with a minimum of ten participants, as statistical power is limited to detect differences in small groups.

Training Evaluation Results

Training on Screening and Assessment

The goal of the screening and assessment training was to increase knowledge about depression among caregivers, to improve confidence for assessing depression and making appropriate referrals, and to enhance service coordinators' ability to make referrals. Alliance service coordinators and supervisors attended sessions that utilized both a traditional classroom lecture format and interactive activities designed to increase comfort with screening and referral processes and promote interactions between training participants. The training also addressed culture and depression (i.e., perception of depression, stigma, treatment services) to facilitate discussion on the issue. Fifty-eight staff participated in the training evaluation. Both the pre- and post-training surveys covered information about caregiver depression and child development, and working with dual-risk families (Figure A.1).

Training participants represented a range of professional degrees and specialties. More than two-thirds reported a bachelor's degree, and slightly less than a third reported a master's degree. The most common areas of study among those with bachelor's and master's degrees were child development and psychology; but a wide variety of additional relevant areas were also represented (e.g., family studies, education, etc.). The remaining participants reported specialty degrees (e.g., a master's in social work or a nursing degree). More than 95 percent of participants reported previous experience with infants and toddlers, and nearly 70 percent reported prior work with preschool children.

As a result of the training on screening and assessment, Alliance staff demonstrated a statistically significant gain in perceived knowledge about the link between caregiver depression and childhood development (t [56]=5.10, p<.01). Furthermore, a four-item quiz administered before and after the training also suggested improvements in knowledge of the prevalence of depression and developmental delays (Table A.2).

Training participants also demonstrated significant improvement in most of their beliefs about screening and assessment (Table A.3).

A ten-item scale was administered before and after the screening and assessment training to measure participants' comfort in addressing depression and behavioral health problems and

Table A.2
Knowledge of Depression and Developmental Delays

Item (Correct Answer in Parentheses)	Percent Correct	
	Pre	Post
Estimated number of children with a depressed caregiver in the United States (15 million)	43	88
Estimated number of children with a depressed caregiver in Allegheny County (about 14,000)	45	86
The Alliance receives more that 3,000 referrals for children at risk for developmental delays (True)	97	95
Risk for depression for mothers of premature babies (twice the rate of mothers of full-term babies)	57	84

Figure A.1
Screening and Assessment Training: Pre- and Post-Test Items

ID # ________

Helping Families Raise Healthy Children Training Assessment

As part of the Helping Families Raise Healthy Children initiative, the Alliance for Infants and Toddlers is inviting you to participate in an evaluation of the training you are attending today. We would like to learn more about the impact of this training session on staff knowledge, attitudes, and practices. The goal of this part of the evaluation is to identify useful aspects of training as well as training gaps for future initiative efforts.

If you choose to participate in the training evaluation, you will complete a short questionnaire prior to today's training and immediately after the training. These questionnaires will ask about your knowledge, attitudes, and behaviors related to working with families affected by both parental depression and early childhood developmental delays (hereafter referred to as "dual-risk families"). You will also be asked to provide your email address so that The Alliance can contact you within two months after this training to complete a third web-based questionnaire. This third questionnaire will include some questions about if and how you have incorporated lessons from the training into your daily practices related to helping dual-risk families.

Your participation is completely voluntary and you have the option to withdraw at any time. All questionnaire answers will be kept confidential. Questionnaires will only have a number on them, and contact lists linking your name with the identification numbers will be kept in a separate, secure file. We will destroy these contact lists after the project is completed. Only project staff will have access to this data. We will only share aggregate findings from these questionnaires in reports on the Helping Families Raise Healthy Children initiative and in communications with our partners, including the RAND Corporation and Community Care Behavioral Health Organization.

If you have any questions about this project, you may contact Patricia Schake at Community Care at schakepl@ccbh.com.

If you choose to participate, please sign below and complete the contact sheet for follow-up on the next page.

________________________ ________________
Print Name Date

____
Signature

MCHC4 Training Pre-Post Survey
SC Training November 17-19, 2009

Figure A.1—Continued

ID # _____

Helping Families Raise Healthy Children Training Evaluation
Contact Form for 2 Month Follow-Up with Trainees

Name: _____

Organization: _____

Address: _____

_____

_____

Email Address: _____

Preferred Phone Number: _____

Alternative Phone Number: _____

Figure A.1—Continued

ID # _____

Helping Families Raise Healthy Children Service Coordination Screening, Referral, and Assessment Training (Pre-Training)

Before we begin this training session, please take 10 minutes to complete this short pre-survey. Thank you.

A.	**Background Information**

1.   What is your professional specialty?   *(Circle One)*

    a.   Early Intervention Service Coordinator 1
    b.   Social worker 2
    c.   Clinical Social Worker... 3
    d.   Marriage and Family Therapist.. 4
    e.   School Psychologist.. 5
    f.   Clinical Psychologist... 6
    g.   Psychiatrist.. 7
    h.   Nursing.. 8
    i.   Other (*specify*: _____)............ 9

2.   What is your professional degree or certification?   *(Circle All That Apply)*

    a.   BA/BS in (specify_____)............. 1
    b.   MA/MS in (specify_____)............. 2
    c.   MSW.. 3
    d.   LCSW... 4
    e.   MS Psychology.. 5
    f.   Ph.D., Psychology... 6
    g.   MFCC / MFT.. 7
    h.   RN or BSN.. 8
    i.   Other (*specify*: _____)............. 9

3.   Do you have experience with the following types of therapy?   *(Circle All That Apply)*

    a.   Individual therapy for children 1
    b.   Group therapy for children 2
    c.   Individual therapy for parents... 3
    d.   Group therapy for parents.. 4
    e.   Family-centered interventions 5
    f.   Other (*specify*: _____) 6

Figure A.1—Continued

ID # _____

4. With which age groups have you worked with?   *(Circle All That Apply)*

    a. Infants and toddlers 1
    b. Preschool age.. 2
    c. Elementary school-aged 3
    d. Middle school-aged 4
    e. High school-aged.. 5
    f. Adult.. 6
    g. Elderly 7

B.   Information about Caregiver Depression and Child Development

5. How much do you feel you already know about the link between caregiver depression and childhood development?

    A great deal..1
    Some..2
    A little..3
    Nothing at all 4

6. All of the options below are symptoms of depression; which pair represents the two that *primarily* characterize depression?

    Guilt and fatigue 1
    Loss of appetite and sadness 2
    Sleep problems and loss of appetite 3
    Sadness and lack of interest/pleasure in most activities 4
    Suicidal thoughts and sleep problems 5

7. Which of the following statements is **true**? Compared to women, men are . . .

    twice as likely to exhibit symptoms of depression 1
    more likely to report guilt as a symptom of depression 2
    more likely to report irritability as a symptom of depression 3

8. At this point (prior to Service Coordination training), to what degree do you consider yourself able to address the behavioral health needs of the *caregivers* of the children you serve? *(Circle one)*

    A great deal... 1
    Somewhat 2
    A little.. 3
    Not at all 4

Figure A.1—Continued

ID # _____

9.   Caregiver depression poses a big enough risk to healthy childhood development that children with a caregiver(s) at risk for depression should be eligible for evaluation by The Alliance.

       Strongly Agree... 1
       Agree 2
       Neutral 3
       Disagree... 4
       Strongly Disagree 5

10.   There is good coordination between the adult behavioral health and the early intervention systems of care.

       Strongly Agree... 1
       Agree 2
       Neutral 3
       Disagree... 4
       Strongly Disagree 5

11.   One of my responsibilities as a Service Coordinator is to screen the caregiver(s) of the children I serve for depression and other behavioral health issues.

       Strongly Agree... 1
       Agree 2
       Neutral 3
       Disagree... 4
       Strongly Disagree 5

12.   If I identify a caregiver at risk for depression, I can refer that caregiver to appropriate behavioral health services.

       Strongly Agree... 1
       Agree 2
       Neutral 3
       Disagree... 4
       Strongly Disagree 5

13.   I am well-aware of the services that the Re:solve Crisis Network can offer to families.

       Strongly Agree... 1
       Agree 2
       Neutral 3
       Disagree... 4
       Strongly Disagree 5

Figure A.1—Continued

ID # _____

14. The four key steps in a service coordinator's response to a dual-risk family are:

Listen, problem solve, affirm strengths, and review options................................1
Listen, document, file notes, and follow-up 2
Problem solve, give advice, review options, and file notes...................................3

C.   Working with Dual-Risk Families

15.   Imagine that today you will see a 2 year old together with his mother, and that the mother is severely depressed. In the session that you will have today, please circle how you would rate your ability/comfort with <u>interacting with this family</u>: *very comfortable*, *somewhat comfortable*, *a little comfortable*, or *not comfortable at all*.

Statement I would feel comfortable to...	*Circle one*			
	Very comfortable	Somewhat comfortable	A little comfortable	Not comfortable at all
a. Use an evidence-based tool to measure symptoms of depression	4	3	2	1
b. Talk with the caregiver about their symptoms of depression	4	3	2	1
c. Talk with the caregiver about the potential impact of depression on child development	4	3	2	1
d. Ask the caregiver about suicidal ideation	4	3	2	1
e. Ask the caregiver about relationship safety/domestic violence (assuming the caregiver's partner is not present)	4	3	2	1
f. Do further assessment of the caregiver's stress	4	3	2	1
g. Do further assessment of the caregiver's physical health	4	3	2	1
h. Make recommendations about behavioral health services for the caregiver	4	3	2	1
i. Make referrals to appropriate behavioral health services for the caregiver	4	3	2	1
j. Address caregiver concerns about engaging in behavioral health treatment	4	3	2	1
k. Call the Re:solve crisis network, if needed, to learn of additional options for this family	4	3	2	1

Figure A.1—Continued

ID # _____

16. How confident are you that you can ask caregivers of the children you serve about depression?

Not at all confident 1
A little confident... 2
Somewhat confident 3
Very confident... 4
Completely confident 5

17. How confident are you that you can screen caregivers of the children you serve for depression using an evidence-based tool?

Not at all confident 1
A little confident... 2
Somewhat confident 3
Very confident... 4
Completely confident 5

18. How confident are you that you can refer the caregivers of the children you serve to adult behavioral health providers?

Not at all confident 1
A little confident... 2
Somewhat confident 3
Very confident... 4
Completely confident 5

19. How confident are you that you can refer the families you serve to behavioral health providers for family-centered interventions?

Not at all confident 1
A little confident... 2
Somewhat confident 3
Very confident... 4
Completely confident 5

20. How confident are you that you can talk to a case manager from Community Care to identity behavioral health providers for the families that you serve?

Not at all confident 1
A little confident... 2
Somewhat confident 3
Very confident... 4
Completely confident 5

Figure A.1—Continued

ID # ________

PRE-TRAINING:

STOP HERE

PLEASE CLOSE THE SURVEY PACKET NOW.

MCHC4 Training Pre-Post Survey
SC SAR Training February 16-19, 2009

Figure A.1—Continued

ID # _____

Helping Families Raise Healthy Children Service Coordination Training (Post-Training)

Now that you have completed the training session, please take 10 minutes to complete this short post-survey. Thank you.

A.	Training

1. After this training, how much do you feel you now know about the link between caregiver depression and childhood development?

   A great deal... 1
   Some 2
   A little... 3
   Nothing at all 4

2. What aspects of the training (e.g., content, how training delivered) did you like?

   _____

   _____

   _____

3. What aspects of the training (e.g., content, how training delivered) would you change?

   _____

   _____

   _____

4. What did you learn in this training that you will use in your work?

   _____

   _____

   _____

   _____

Figure A.1—Continued

ID # _____

5.   Are there things presented in this training that you would not use in your work? If so, what and why not?

_____

_____

_____

_____

B.   Helping Families Raise Healthy Children Next Steps

6. Now that you have completed this training, how confident are you that you can ask caregivers of the children you serve about depression?

Not at all confident 1
A little confident.. 2
Somewhat confident 3
Very confident 4
Completely confident 5

7.   Now that you have completed this training, how confident are you that you can screen caregivers of the children you serve for depression using an evidence-based tool?

Not at all confident 1
A little confident.. 2
Somewhat confident 3
Very confident 4
Completely confident 5

8.   Now that you have completed this training, how confident are you that you can refer the caregivers of the children you serve to adult behavioral health providers?

Not at all confident 1
A little confident.. 2
Somewhat confident 3
Very confident 4
Completely confident 5

Figure A.1—Continued

ID # _____

9.   Now that you have completed this training, how confident are you that you can refer the families you serve to behavioral health providers for family-centered interventions?

       Not at all confident 1
       A little confident.. 2
       Somewhat confident 3
       Very confident 4
       Completely confident 5

10.   Now that you have completed this training, how confident are you that you can talk to a case manager from Community Care to identity behavioral health providers for the families that you serve?

       Not at all confident 1
       A little confident.. 2
       Somewhat confident 3
       Very confident 4
       Completely confident 5

C.   Information about Caregiver Depression and Child Development

11.   All of the options below are symptoms of depression; which pair represents the two that *primarily* characterize depression?

       Guilt and fatigue 1
       Loss of appetite and sadness 2
       Sleep problems and loss of appetite 3
       Sadness and lack of interest/pleasure in most activities 4
       Suicidal thoughts and sleep problems 5

12.   Which of the following statements is **true**? Compared to women, men are . . .

       twice as likely to exhibit symptoms of depression 1
       more likely to report guilt as a symptom of depression 2
       more likely to report irritability as a symptom of depression 3

13.   At this point, to what degree do you consider yourself able to address the behavioral health needs of the *caregivers* of the children you serve? *(Circle one)*

       A great deal.. 1
       Somewhat 2
       A little... 3
       Not at all 4

Figure A.1—Continued

ID # _____

14. Caregiver depression poses a big enough risk to healthy childhood development that children with a caregiver(s) at risk for depression should be eligible for evaluation by The Alliance.

    Strongly Agree 1
    Agree 2
    Neutral 3
    Disagree 4
    Strongly Disagree 5

15. There is good coordination between the adult behavioral health and the early intervention systems of care.

    Strongly Agree 1
    Agree 2
    Neutral 3
    Disagree 4
    Strongly Disagree 5

16. One of my responsibilities as a Service Coordinator is to screen the caregiver(s) of the children I serve for depression and other behavioral health issues.

    Strongly Agree 1
    Agree 2
    Neutral 3
    Disagree 4
    Strongly Disagree 5

17. If I identify a caregiver at risk for depression, I can refer that caregiver to appropriate behavioral health services.

    Strongly Agree 1
    Agree 2
    Neutral 3
    Disagree 4
    Strongly Disagree 5

18. I am well-aware of the services that the Re:solve Crisis Network can offer to families.

    Strongly Agree 1
    Agree 2
    Neutral 3
    Disagree 4
    Strongly Disagree 5

Figure A.1—Continued

ID # _____

19. The four key steps in a service coordinator's response to a dual-risk family are:

Listen, problem solve, affirm strengths, and review options 1
Listen, document, file notes, and follow-up 2
Problem solve, give advice, review options, and file notes 3

20. Imagine that today you will see a 2 year old together with his mother, and that the mother is severely depressed. In the session that you will have today, please circle how you would rate your ability/comfort with interacting with this family: *very comfortable*, *somewhat comfortable*, *a little comfortable*, or *not comfortable at all*.

Statement I would feel comfortable to...	Circle one			
	Very comfortable	Somewhat comfortable	A little comfortable	Not comfortable at all
l. Use an evidence-based tool to measure symptoms of depression	4	3	2	1
m. Talk with the caregiver about their symptoms of depression	4	3	2	1
n. Talk with the caregiver about the potential impact of depression on child development	4	3	2	1
o. Ask the caregiver about suicidal ideation	4	3	2	1
p. Ask the caregiver about relationship safety/domestic violence (assuming the caregiver's partner is not present)	4	3	2	1
q. Do further assessment of the caregiver's stress	4	3	2	1
r. Do further assessment of the caregiver's physical health	4	3	2	1
s. Make recommendations about behavioral health services for the caregiver	4	3	2	1
t. Make referrals to appropriate behavioral health services for the caregiver	4	3	2	1
u. Address caregiver concerns about engaging in behavioral health treatment	4	3	2	1
v. Call the Re:solve crisis network, if needed, to learn of additional options for this family	4	3	2	1

Table A.3
Beliefs About Screening and Assessment

Belief	Pre	Post	Significance Level
At this point, to what degree do you consider yourself able to address the behavioral health needs of the caregivers of the children you serve?	3.30	3.91	<.01
Caregiver depression poses a big enough risk to healthy childhood development that children with a caregiver(or caregivers) at risk for depression should be eligible for evaluation by The Alliance.	4.18	4.30	n.s.
There is good coordination between the adult behavioral health and the early intervention systems of care.	2.42	3.11	<.01
One of my responsibilities as a service coordinator is to screen the caregiver(s) of the children I serve for depression and other behavioral health issues.	3.29	4.05	<.01
If I identify a caregiver as being at risk for depression, I can refer that caregiver to appropriate behavioral health services.	3.61	3.95	<.01

NOTE: 1=strongly disagree, 5=strongly agree; except for the first item, which ranged from 1=not at all to 4=a great deal; n.s.=non-significant.

assisting caregivers in obtaining appropriate treatment (Figure A.1). Analysis of this scale indicated increased comfort in performing these activities after the training session was completed (t [56]=–5.31, p<.01).

Additional items assessed whether the training was effective in improving participants' confidence in their abilities to ask caregivers about depression, screen caregivers with an evidence-based tool, refer caregivers to behavioral health providers, and refer families to providers for relationship-based interventions. Paired t-tests on these items indicated significant improvements in trainees' confidence in each of these domains (p's<.01). Trainees did not report significant changes in their ability to discuss potential behavioral health providers with case managers from Community Care; however, the pre-training mean (m=3.26) suggested that most participants were somewhat to very confident that they could engage with case managers before the training.

Training on Referrals

The goal of the referral training was to increase participants' ability to make referrals. Forty-three staff members from The Alliance (service coordinators and supervisors) participated in the evaluation of this training.

Both the pre- and post-training surveys for the referral trainings covered information about caregiver depression and child development, and about working with dual-risk families (Figure A.2).

Participants in the training represented a range of education and professional backgrounds. Nearly three quarters of training participants reported a bachelor's degree. The majority of the remaining participants reported a master's degree; others reported a specialty degree (e.g., a master's in social work) or did not report their professional education. Almost 90 percent of training participants reported previous experience with infants and toddlers, and nearly 75 percent reported prior work with preschool children.

On average, participants reported that they knew "some" about the link between caregiver depression and childhood development. This did not change from the pre-training assessment to the post-training assessment. A two-item quiz administered before and after

Figure A.2
Referral Training: Pre- and Post-Test Items

ID # ________

Helping Families Raise Healthy Children Training Assessment

As part of the Helping Families Raise Healthy Children initiative, the Alliance for Infants and Toddlers is inviting you to participate in an evaluation of the training you are attending today. We would like to learn more about the impact of this training session on staff knowledge, attitudes, and practices. The goal of this part of the evaluation is to identify useful aspects of training as well as training gaps for future initiative efforts.

If you choose to participate in the training evaluation, you will complete a short questionnaire prior to today's training and immediately after the training. These questionnaires will ask about your knowledge, attitudes, and behaviors related to working with families affected by both parental depression and early childhood developmental delays (hereafter referred to as "dual-risk families"). You will also be asked to provide your email address so that The Alliance can contact you within two months after this training to complete a third web-based questionnaire. This third questionnaire will include some questions about if and how you have incorporated lessons from the training into your daily practices related to helping dual-risk families.

Your participation is completely voluntary and you have the option to withdraw at any time. All questionnaire answers will be kept confidential. Questionnaires will only have a number on them, and contact lists linking your name with the identification numbers will be kept in a separate, secure file. We will destroy these contact lists after the project is completed. Only project staff will have access to this data. We will only share aggregate findings from these questionnaires in reports on the Helping Families Raise Healthy Children initiative and in communications with our partners, including the RAND Corporation and Community Care Behavioral Health Organization.

If you have any questions about this project, you may contact Patricia Schake at Community Care at schakepl@ccbh.com.

If you choose to participate, please sign below and complete the contact sheet for follow-up on the next page.

______________________________ ______________________
Print Name Date

____
Signature

MCHC4 Training Pre-Post Survey
SC Training November 17-19, 2009

Figure A.2—Continued

ID # ________

Helping Families Raise Healthy Children Training Evaluation
Contact Form for 2 Month Follow-Up with Trainees

Name: ______________________________

Organization: ______________________________

Address: ______________________________

____

____

Email Address: ______________________________

Preferred Phone Number: ______________________________

Alternative Phone Number: ______________________________

MCHC4 Training Pre-Post Survey
SC Training November 17-19, 2009

Figure A.2—Continued

ID # _____

Helping Families Raise Healthy Children Service Coordination Training (Pre-Training)

Before we begin this training session, please take 10 minutes to complete this short pre-survey. Thank you.

A.	**Background Information**

1.   What is your professional specialty?   *(Circle One)*

    a.   Early Intervention Service Coordinator 1
    b.   Social worker 2
    c.   Clinical Social Worker... 3
    d.   Marriage and Family Therapist... 4
    e.   School Psychologist.. 5
    f.   Clinical Psychologist... 6
    g.   Psychiatrist.. 7
    h.   Nursing.. 8
    i.   Other (*specify*: _____)........... 9

2.   What is your professional degree or certification?   *(Circle All That Apply)*

    a.   BA/BS in (specify_____).............. 1
    b.   MA/MS in (specify_____).............. 2
    c.   MSW... 3
    d.   LCSW.. 4
    e.   MS Psychology... 5
    f.   Ph.D., Psychology.. 6
    g.   MFCC / MFT.. 7
    h.   RN or BSN.. 8
    i.   Other (*specify*: _____).............. 9

3.   Do you have experience with the following types of therapy?   *(Circle All That Apply)*

    a.   Individual therapy for children 1
    b.   Group therapy for children 2
    c.   Individual therapy for parents.. 3
    d.   Group therapy for parents... 4
    e.   Family-centered interventions 5
    f.   Other (*specify*: _____) 6

Figure A.2—Continued

ID # _____

4. With which age groups have you worked with?   *(Circle All That Apply)*

    a.   Infants and toddlers 1
    b.   Preschool age... 2
    c.   Elementary school-aged 3
    d.   Middle school-aged 4
    e.   High school-aged... 5
    f.   Adult... 6
    g.   Elderly 7

B.   Information about Caregiver Depression and Child Development

5. How much do you feel you already know about the link between caregiver depression and childhood development?

    A great deal..1
    Some..2
    A little...3
    Nothing at all 4

6. Each year, the estimated number of children living with a caregiver with depression in the United States is:

    1 million.. 1
    5 million.. 2
    15 million.. 3
    30 million.. 4
    60 million.. 5

7. Each year, the estimated number of children living with a caregiver with depression in Allegheny County is:

    About 1000 1
    About 14,000 2
    About 20,000 3
    About 50,000 4

8. **True or False**: Each year, The Alliance for Infants and Toddlers receives more than 3,000 referrals for children at risk for developmental delays

    True.. 1
    False.. 2

Figure A.2—Continued

ID # _____

9. Which of the following statements is **true**? Compared to mothers of full-term babies, mothers of premature babies are . . .

twice as likely to exhibit symptoms of depression 1
four times as likely to exhibit symptoms of depression 2
no more likely to exhibit symptoms of depression 3

10. At this point (prior to Service Coordination training), to what degree do you consider yourself able to address the behavioral health needs of the *caregivers* of the children you serve? *(Circle one)*

A great deal... 1
Somewhat 2
A little.. 3
Not at all 4

11. Caregiver depression poses a big enough risk to healthy childhood development that children with a caregiver(s) at risk for depression should be eligible for evaluation by The Alliance.

Strongly Agree... 1
Agree 2
Neutral 3
Disagree.. 4
Strongly Disagree 5

12. There is good coordination between the adult behavioral health and the early intervention systems of care.

Strongly Agree... 1
Agree 2
Neutral 3
Disagree.. 4
Strongly Disagree 5

13. One of my responsibilities as a Service Coordinator is to screen the caregiver(s) of the children I serve for depression and other behavioral health issues.

Strongly Agree... 1
Agree 2
Neutral 3
Disagree.. 4
Strongly Disagree 5

Figure A.2—Continued

14.   If I identify a caregiver at risk for depression, I can refer that caregiver to appropriate behavioral health services.

        Strongly Agree 1
        Agree 2
        Neutral 3
        Disagree 4
        Strongly Disagree 5

C.   Working with Dual-Risk Families

15.   Imagine that today you will see a 2 year old together with his mother, and that the mother is severely depressed. In the session that you will have today, please circle how you would rate your ability/comfort with <u>interacting with this family</u>: *very comfortable*, *somewhat comfortable*, *a little comfortable*, or *not comfortable at all*.

Statement I would feel comfortable to…	*Circle one*			
	Very comfortable	Somewhat comfortable	A little comfortable	Not comfortable at all
a. Use an evidence-based tool to measure symptoms of depression	4	3	2	1
b. Talk with the caregiver about their symptoms of depression	4	3	2	1
c. Talk with the caregiver about the potential impact of depression on child development	4	3	2	1
d. Ask the caregiver about suicidal ideation	4	3	2	1
e. Ask the caregiver about relationship safety/domestic violence (assuming the caregiver's partner is not present)	4	3	2	1
f. Do further assessment of the caregiver's stress	4	3	2	1
g. Do further assessment of the caregiver's physical health	4	3	2	1
h. Make recommendations about behavioral health services for the caregiver	4	3	2	1
i. Make referrals to appropriate behavioral health services for the caregiver	4	3	2	1
j. Address caregiver concerns about engaging in behavioral health treatment	4	3	2	1

Figure A.2—Continued

ID # _____

16. How confident are you that you can ask caregivers of the children you serve about depression?

Not at all confident 1
A little confident... 2
Somewhat confident 3
Very confident.. 4
Completely confident 5

17. How confident are you that you can screen caregivers of the children you serve for depression using an evidence-based tool?

Not at all confident 1
A little confident... 2
Somewhat confident 3
Very confident.. 4
Completely confident 5

18. How confident are you that you can refer the caregivers of the children you serve to adult behavioral health providers?

Not at all confident 1
A little confident... 2
Somewhat confident 3
Very confident.. 4
Completely confident 5

19. How confident are you that you can refer the families you serve to behavioral health providers for family-centered interventions?

Not at all confident 1
A little confident... 2
Somewhat confident 3
Very confident.. 4
Completely confident 5

20. How confident are you that you can talk to a case manager from Community Care to identity behavioral health providers for the families that you serve?

Not at all confident 1
A little confident... 2
Somewhat confident 3
Very confident.. 4
Completely confident 5

Figure A.2—Continued

ID # _____

PRE-TRAINING:

STOP HERE

PLEASE CLOSE THE SURVEY PACKET NOW.

Figure A.2—Continued

ID # ________

Helping Families Raise Healthy Children Service Coordination Training (Post-Training)

Now that you have completed the training session, please take 10 minutes to complete this short post-survey. Thank you.

A. Training

1. After this training, how much do you feel you now know about the link between caregiver depression and childhood development?

A great deal 1
Some 2
A little 3
Nothing at all 4

2. What aspects of the training (e.g., content, how training delivered) did you like?

____

____

____

3. What aspects of the training (e.g., content, how training delivered) would you change?

____

____

____

4. What did you learn in this training that you will use in your work?

____

____

____

____

MCHC4 Training Pre-Post Survey
SC Training November 17-19, 2009

Figure A.2—Continued

ID # _____

5. Are there things presented in this training that you would not use in your work? If so, what and why not?

_____

_____

_____

_____

B.   Helping Families Raise Healthy Children Next Steps

6. Now that you have completed this training, how confident are you that you can ask caregivers of the children you serve about depression?

Not at all confident 1
A little confident.. 2
Somewhat confident 3
Very confident 4
Completely confident 5

7. Now that you have completed this training, how confident are you that you can screen caregivers of the children you serve for depression using an evidence-based tool?

Not at all confident 1
A little confident.. 2
Somewhat confident 3
Very confident 4
Completely confident 5

8. Now that you have completed this training, how confident are you that you can refer the caregivers of the children you serve to adult behavioral health providers?

Not at all confident 1
A little confident.. 2
Somewhat confident 3
Very confident 4
Completely confident 5

Figure A.2—Continued

ID # _____

9.   Now that you have completed this training, how confident are you that you can refer the families you serve to behavioral health providers for family-centered interventions?

    Not at all confident 1
    A little confident.. 2
    Somewhat confident 3
    Very confident 4
    Completely confident 5

10.   Now that you have completed this training, how confident are you that you can talk to a case manager from Community Care to identity behavioral health providers for the families that you serve?

    Not at all confident 1
    A little confident.. 2
    Somewhat confident 3
    Very confident 4
    Completely confident 5

C.   Information about Caregiver Depression and Child Development

11.   Each year, the estimated number of children living with a caregiver with depression in the United States is:

    1 million.. 1
    5 million.. 2
    15 million.. 3
    30 million.. 4
    60 million.. 5

12.   Each year, the estimated number of children living with a caregiver with depression in Allegheny County is:

    About 1000 1
    About 14,000 2
    About 20,000 3
    About 50,000 4

13.   **True or False**: Each year, The Alliance for Infants and Toddlers receives more than 3,000 referrals for children at risk for developmental delays

    True.. 1
    False... 2

Figure A.2—Continued

ID # _____

14. Which of the following statements is **true**? Compared to mothers of full-term babies, mothers of premature babies are . . .

    twice as likely to exhibit symptoms of depression 1
    four times as likely to exhibit symptoms of depression 2
    no more likely to exhibit symptoms of depression 3

15. At this point, to what degree do you consider yourself able to address the behavioral health needs of the *caregivers* of the children you serve? *(Circle one)*

    A great deal.. 1
    Somewhat 2
    A little 3
    Not at all 4

16. Caregiver depression poses a big enough risk to healthy childhood development that children with a caregiver(s) at risk for depression should be eligible for evaluation by The Alliance.

    Strongly Agree.. 1
    Agree 2
    Neutral 3
    Disagree.. 4
    Strongly Disagree 5

17. There is good coordination between the adult behavioral health and the early intervention systems of care.

    Strongly Agree.. 1
    Agree 2
    Neutral 3
    Disagree.. 4
    Strongly Disagree 5

18. One of my responsibilities as a Service Coordinator is to screen the caregiver(s) of the children I serve for depression and other behavioral health issues.

    Strongly Agree.. 1
    Agree 2
    Neutral 3
    Disagree.. 4
    Strongly Disagree 5

Figure A.2—Continued

ID # _____

19.   If I identify a caregiver at risk for depression, I can refer that caregiver to appropriate behavioral health services.

Strongly Agree.. 1
Agree 2
Neutral 3
Disagree.. 4
Strongly Disagree 5

20.   Imagine that today you will see a 2 year old together with his mother, and that the mother is severely depressed. In the session that you will have today, please circle how you would rate your ability/comfort with <u>interacting with this family</u>: *very comfortable, somewhat comfortable, a little comfortable*, or *not comfortable at all*.

Statement **I would feel comfortable to…**	*Circle one*			
	Very comfortable	Somewhat comfortable	A little comfortable	Not comfortable at all
k. Use an evidence-based tool to measure symptoms of depression	4	3	2	1
l. Talk with the caregiver about their symptoms of depression	4	3	2	1
m. Talk with the caregiver about the potential impact of depression on child development	4	3	2	1
n. Ask the caregiver about suicidal ideation	4	3	2	1
o. Ask the caregiver about relationship safety/domestic violence (assuming the caregiver's partner is not present)	4	3	2	1
p. Do further assessment of the caregiver's stress	4	3	2	1
q. Do further assessment of the caregiver's physical health	4	3	2	1
r. Make recommendations about behavioral health services for the caregiver	4	3	2	1
s. Make referrals to appropriate behavioral health services for the caregiver	4	3	2	1
t. Address caregiver concerns about engaging in behavioral health treatment	4	3	2	1

the training suggests changes in knowledge about depression, but not in the expected direction (Table A.4). For the first item, it may be that a more thorough understanding of depression resulted in the respondents questioning what qualified as the "primary" symptoms. More broadly, since this training was focused on providing Alliance service coordinators with details on the referral process, it may not have been the best setting for imparting more general information about depression.

Alliance staff also demonstrated significant changes in all but one of their beliefs about screening and assessment (Table A.5). For these items, an increase in score represented improvement on the measure.

A ten-item scale was administered before and after the training to assess participants' comfort in assessing depression and behavioral health problems and assisting caregivers in obtaining appropriate treatment (Figure A.2). Analysis of this scale indicated increased comfort in performing these activities after the training session was completed (paired t-test, t[39]= −6.10, p<.01). The specific items relevant to referrals were especially important to this training, which focused on the referral process (Table A.6). Paired t-tests on these items indicated significant improvements in trainees' confidence in each of these domains (p's<.01). For each of these items, the training participants reported increased comfort with the referral process; an increase in score represented improvement on the measure.

Additional items assessed whether the training was effective in improving participants' confidence about asking caregivers about depression, screening caregivers with an evidence-

Table A.4
Knowledge About Depression

	Percent Correct	
Item	Pre	Post
Primary symptoms of depression (sadness and lack of interest/pleasure in most activities)	81	65
Difference in symptoms between men and women (men more likely to report irritability as a symptom of depression)	63	53

Table A.5
Beliefs About Screening and Assessment

Belief	Pre	Post	Significance Level
At this point, to what degree do you consider yourself able to address the behavioral health needs of the caregivers of the children you serve?	3.44	4.02	<.01
Caregiver depression poses a big enough risk to healthy childhood development that children with a caregiver(s) at risk for depression should be eligible for evaluation by The Alliance.	3.92	3.87	n.s.
There is good coordination between the adult behavioral health and the early intervention systems of care.	2.61	3.32	<.01
One of my responsibilities as a Service Coordinator is to screen the caregiver(s) of the children I serve for depression and other behavioral health issues.	3.20	3.66	<.01
If I identify a caregiver at risk for depression, I can refer that caregiver to appropriate behavioral health services.	3.30	3.97	<.01
I am well-aware of the services that the Re:solve Crisis Network can offer to families.	2.85	4.25	<.01

NOTE. 1=strongly disagree; 5=strongly agree; except for the first item, which ranged from 1=not at all to 4=a great deal. n.s.=not statistically significant.

Table A.6
Comfort Level with Referral Process

Item	Pre	Post	Significance Level
Make recommendations about behavioral health services for the caregiver	2.48	2.95	<.01
Make referrals to appropriate behavioral health services for the caregiver	2.59	3.13	<.01
Address caregiver concerns about engaging in behavioral health treatment	2.53	3.00	<.01
Call the Re:solve crisis network, if needed, to learn of additional options for this family	2.74	3.33	<.01

NOTE: 1=not at all comfortable, 4=very comfortable.

based tool, referring caregivers to behavioral health providers, referring families to providers for relationship-based interventions, and asking Community Care care-managers to identify behavioral health providers for families. Paired t-tests indicated significant improvements in trainees' confidence in each of these domains (p's<.01).

Training on Infant Mental Health and Relationship-Based Treatment

The goal of this community-based training was to provide participants with an overview of infant mental health and relationship-based treatment. Responses to an evaluation survey were obtained from 108 participants. Both the pre- and post-training surveys for this training covered information about infant mental health and attachment and working with dual-risk families (Figure A.3).

Individuals participating in the training represented a range of educational and professional backgrounds. Participants included early intervention service coordinators, social workers, nurses, psychologists, and therapists, among others. Just over a third of training participants reported a bachelor's degree, just under a third reported a master's degree, and the remaining participants reported specialty degrees/certifications (e.g., those with a master's in social work, licensed clinical social workers, registered nurses or those with a bachelor's degree in nursing) or identified their training as "other." Almost 90 percent of training participants reported previous experience with infants and toddlers and more than 80 percent of them reported prior work with preschool children.

Perceived knowledge about infant mental health, infant-caregiver attachment, and the neurobiological basis of infant-caregiver attachment all improved from pre-training to post-training (p's<.01). The results of a two-item quiz administered before and after the training are provided in Table A.7.

Service coordinators also demonstrated significant changes in their beliefs about infant mental health and attachment (Table A.8). For these items, an increase in score represented improvement on the measure.

Table A.7
Knowledge of Infant Mental Health and Infant-Caregiver Attachment

Item (Correct Answer Is in Parentheses)	Percent Correct	
	Pre	Post
Brain development is most rapid (during the first three years of life)	51	85
The estimated prevalence of depression among caregivers of children with developmental delays is (40 percent)	34	58

Figure A.3
Infant Mental Health Training: Pre- and Post-Test Items

ID # ________

Helping Families Raise Healthy Children Training Assessment

As part of the Helping Families Raise Healthy Children initiative, the Alliance for Infants and Toddlers is inviting you to participate in an evaluation of the training you are attending today. We would like to learn more about the impact of this training session on staff knowledge, attitudes, and practices. The goal of this part of the evaluation is to identify useful aspects of training as well as training gaps for future initiative efforts.

If you choose to participate in the training evaluation, you will complete a short questionnaire prior to today's training and immediately after the training. These questionnaires will ask about your knowledge, attitudes, and behaviors related to infant mental health and to working with families affected by both parental depression and early childhood developmental delays (hereafter referred to as "dual-risk families"). You will also be asked to provide your email address so that The Alliance can contact you within two months after this training to complete a third web-based questionnaire. This third questionnaire will include some questions about if and how you have incorporated lessons from the training into your daily practices related to helping dual-risk families.

Your participation is completely voluntary and you have the option to withdraw at any time. All questionnaire answers will be kept confidential. Questionnaires will only have a number on them, and contact lists linking your name with the identification numbers will be kept in a separate, secure file. We will destroy these contact lists after the project is completed. Only project staff will have access to this data. We will only share aggregate findings from these questionnaires in reports on the Helping Families Raise Healthy Children initiative and in communications with our partners, including the RAND Corporation and Community Care Behavioral Health Organization.

If you have any questions about this project, you may contact Patricia Schake at Community Care at schakepl@ccbh.com.

If you choose to participate, please sign below and complete the contact sheet for follow-up on the next page.

______________________________ ______________________

Print Name Date

____

Signature

MCHC4 Training Pre-Post Survey
IMH Training April 12, 2010

Figure A.3—Continued

ID # ________

Helping Families Raise Healthy Children Training Evaluation
Contact Form for 2 month Follow-Up with Trainees

Name: ______________________________

Organization: ______________________________

Address: ______________________________

____

____

Email Address: ______________________________

Preferred Phone Number: ______________________________

Alternative Phone Number: ______________________________

MCHC4 Training Pre-Post Survey
IMH Training April 12, 2010

Figure A.3—Continued

ID # _____

Helping Families Raise Healthy Children Infant Mental Health Training (Pre-Training)

Before we begin this training session, please take 10 minutes to complete this short pre-survey. Thank you.

A.   Background Information

1.   What is your professional specialty?   *(Circle One)*

    a. Early Intervention Service Coordinator   1
    b. Social worker   2
    c. Clinical Social Worker...   3
    d. Marriage and Family Therapist..   4
    e. School Psychologist..   5
    f. Clinical Psychologist...   6
    g. Psychiatrist...   7
    h. Nursing...   8
    i. Other (*specify*: _____)...........   9

2.   What is your professional degree or certification?   *(Circle All That Apply)*

    a. BA/BS in (specify_____)...............   1
    b. MA/MS in (specify_____)...............   2
    c. MSW..   3
    d. LCSW...   4
    e. MS Psychology..   5
    f. Ph.D., Psychology..   6
    g. MFCC / MFT...   7
    h. RN or BSN..   8
    i. Other (*specify*: _____)...............   9

3.   Do you have experience with the following types of therapy?   *(Circle All That Apply)*

    a. Individual therapy for children   1
    b. Group therapy for children   2
    c. Individual therapy for parents..   3
    d. Group therapy for parents   4
    e. Family-centered interventions   5
    f. Other (*specify*: _____)   6

Figure A.3—Continued

ID # _____

4. With which age groups have you worked with?   *(Circle All That Apply)*

    a.   Infants and toddlers 1
    b.   Preschool age.. 2
    c.   Elementary school-aged 3
    d.   Middle school-aged 4
    e.   High school-aged.. 5
    f.   Adult... 6
    g.   Elderly 7

B.   Information about Infant Mental Health and Attachment

5.   How much do you feel you already know about infant mental health?

        A great deal..1
        Some...2
        A little..3
        Nothing at all 4

6.   How much do you feel you already know about infant-caregiver attachment?

        A great deal..1
        Some...2
        A little..3
        Nothing at all……………………………………..4

7.   How much do you feel you already know about the neurobiological basis of infant-caregiver attachment?

        A great deal..1
        Some...2
        A little..3
        Nothing at all……………………………………..4

8.   Which of the following statements is **true**? Brain development is most rapid . . .

        During the fist year of life 1
        During the first six months of life 2
        During the first three years of life 3

Figure A.3—Continued

ID # ________

9. The estimated prevalence of depression among caregivers of children with developmental delays is . . .

5% 1
25% 2
40% 3
60% 4

10. Stress response and self-regulation are key components of infant mental health.

Strongly Agree........ 1
Agree 2
Neutral 3
Disagree........ 4
Strongly Disagree 5

11. Securely attached infant-caregiver dyads are characterized by more adaptive stress responses and better self-regulation.

Strongly Agree........ 1
Agree 2
Neutral 3
Disagree........ 4
Strongly Disagree 5

12. Several of the symptoms of adult depression can look like suboptimal caregiver attachment behaviors.

Strongly Agree........ 1
Agree 2
Neutral 3
Disagree........ 4
Strongly Disagree 5

MCHC4 Training Pre-Post Survey
IMH Training April 12, 2010

Figure A.3—Continued

ID # _____

C.   Working with Dual-Risk Families

13.   Imagine that today you will see a 2 year old together with his mother, and that the mother is severely depressed. In the session that you will have today, please circle how you would rate your ability/comfort with <u>interacting with this family</u>: *very comfortable*, *somewhat comfortable*, *a little comfortable*, or *not comfortable at all*.

Statement I would feel comfortable to...	*Circle one*			
	Very comfortable	Somewhat comfortable	A little comfortable	Not comfortable at all
a. Talk with the caregiver about their history of abuse or trauma	4	3	2	1
b. Talk with the caregiver about their symptoms of depression	4	3	2	1
c. Engage in joint problem solving with the caregiver	4	3	2	1
d. As the caregiver a series of "joining" questions (e.g., about the child's birth, about their current worries or concerns)	4	3	2	1
e. Conduct a joint observation of the child's behavior with the caregiver	4	3	2	1
f. Do further assessment of the caregiver's stress	4	3	2	1
g. Make recommendations about behavioral health services for the caregiver	4	3	2	1
h. Make referrals to appropriate behavioral health services for the caregiver	4	3	2	1
i. Address caregiver concerns about engaging in behavioral health treatment	4	3	2	1

14.   How confident are you that you can provide early intervention services using a **relationships-based practice** model?

Not at all confident 1
A little confident.. 2
Somewhat confident 3
Very confident 4
Completely confident 5

Figure A.3—Continued

ID # ________

PRE-TRAINING:

STOP HERE

PLEASE CLOSE THE SURVEY PACKET NOW.

MCHC4 Training Pre-Post Survey
IMH Training April 12, 2010

Figure A.3—Continued

ID # ________

Helping Families Raise Healthy Children Service Coordination Training (Post-Training)

Now that you have completed the training session, please take 10 minutes to complete this short post-survey. Thank you.

A. Training

1. What aspects of the training (e.g., content, how training delivered) did you like?

____

____

____

2. What aspects of the training (e.g., content, how training delivered) would you change?

____

____

____

3. What did you learn in this training that you will use in your work?

____

____

____

____

4. Are there things presented in this training that you would not use in your work? If so, what and why not?

____

____

____

____

MCHC4 Training Pre-Post Survey
IMH Training April 12, 2010

Figure A.3—Continued

ID # _____

B.   Helping Families Raise Healthy Children Next Steps

5.   How much do you feel you now know about infant mental health?

A great deal...1
Some...2
A little..3
Nothing at all 4

6.   How much do you feel you now know about infant-caregiver attachment?

A great deal...1
Some...2
A little..3
Nothing at all…………………………..4

7.   How much do you feel you now know about the neurobiological basis of infant-caregiver attachment?

A great deal...1
Some...2
A little..3
Nothing at all…………………………..4

8.   Which of the following statements is **true**? Brain development is most rapid . . .

During the fist year of life 1
During the first six months of life 2
During the first three years of life   3

9.   The estimated prevalence of depression among caregivers of children with developmental delays is . . .

5% 1
25% 2
40% 3
60% …………………………………….4

10.   Stress response and self-regulation are key components of infant mental health.

Strongly Agree.. 1
Agree 2
Neutral 3
Disagree.. 4
Strongly Disagree 5

MCHC4 Training Pre-Post Survey
IMH Training April 12, 2010

Figure A.3—Continued

ID # ________

11. Securely attached infant-caregiver dyads are characterized by more adaptive stress responses and better self-regulation.

    Strongly Agree 1
    Agree 2
    Neutral 3
    Disagree 4
    Strongly Disagree 5

12. Several of the symptoms of adult depression can look like suboptimal caregiver attachment behaviors.

    Strongly Agree 1
    Agree 2
    Neutral 3
    Disagree 4
    Strongly Disagree 5

MCHC4 Training Pre-Post Survey
IMH Training April 12, 2010

Figure A.3—Continued

ID # _____

C.   Working with Dual-Risk Families

13.   Imagine that today you will see a 2 year old together with his mother, and that the mother is severely depressed. In the session that you will have today, please circle how you would rate your ability/comfort with <u>interacting with this family</u>: *very comfortable*, *somewhat comfortable*, *a little comfortable*, or *not comfortable at all*.

Statement I would feel comfortable to...	*Circle one*			
	Very comfortable	Somewhat comfortable	A little comfortable	Not comfortable at all
j. Talk with the caregiver about their history of abuse or trauma	4	3	2	1
k. Talk with the caregiver about their symptoms of depression	4	3	2	1
l. Engage in joint problem solving with the caregiver	4	3	2	1
m. As the caregiver a series of "joining" questions (e.g., about the child's birth, about their current worries or concerns)	4	3	2	1
n. Conduct a joint observation of the child's behavior with the caregiver	4	3	2	1
o. Do further assessment of the caregiver's stress	4	3	2	1
p. Make recommendations about behavioral health services for the caregiver	4	3	2	1
q. Make referrals to appropriate behavioral health services for the caregiver	4	3	2	1
r. Address caregiver concerns about engaging in behavioral health treatment	4	3	2	1

14. Now that you have completed this training, how confident are you that you can provide early intervention services using a **relationships-based practice** model?

Not at all confident 1
A little confident.. 2
Somewhat confident 3
Very confident.. 4

Table A.8
Beliefs About Infant Mental Health and Attachment

Belief	Pre	Post	Significance Level
Stress response and self-regulation are key components of infant mental health.	4.33	4.75	<.01
Securely attached infant-caregiver dyads are characterized by more adaptive stress responses and better self-regulation.	4.34	4.70	<.01
Several of the symptoms of adult depression can look like suboptimal caregiver attachment behaviors.	4.06	4.56	<.01

NOTE: 1=strongly disagree; 5=strongly agree.

A nine-item scale was administered before and after the training to assess participants' comfort in interacting with the family around issues surrounding depression, assessing stress and depression, and making referrals (See Table A.9). Analysis of this scale indicated improvement in participants' comfort in dealing with these issues (paired t-test, t[101]=−8.25, p<.01). Especially important to this training were the items about connecting with the family (Table A.9). For each of these items, the training participants reported increased comfort with the referral process.

The training was also effective in improving participants' confidence about providing early intervention services using a relationships-based practice model (paired t-test, t[89]=−5.55, p<.01).

Training on Specific Relationship-Based Interventions

After attending the initial overview training on infant mental health and relationship-based treatment, early intervention and behavioral service providers received in-depth training in one of three models of well-established techniques employing relationship-based strategies: Nurturing Parenting, Promoting First Relationships, and Partners in Parenting Education. Sessions employed both a traditional classroom lecture format and interactive activities designed to increase comfort in using relationship-based techniques and promote interactions between training participants. Each relationship-based workshop used case discussions and examples from culturally diverse families, which facilitated discussion of culture's impact on the family. Both the pre- and post-training surveys included four items on family-centered practice, including two general questions asked at each of the specific trainings and two questions specific to the relationship-based intervention (Table A.10). The pre-training survey also included the Evidence-Based Practice Attitudes Scale (Aarons, 2004), which was administered to assess provider attitudes toward new practices and approaches to working with families.

Table A.9
Comfort Level Interacting with Families About Depression

Item	Pre	Post	Significance Level
Engage in joint problem-solving with the caregiver	3.17	3.62	<.01
Ask the caregiver a series of "joining" questions (e.g., about the child's birth, about their current worries or concerns)	3.39	3.71	<.01
Conduct a joint observation of the child's behavior with the caregiver	3.33	3.60	<.01

NOTE: 1=not at all comfortable, 4=very comfortable.

Table A.10
Relationship-Based Intervention Training: Pre- and Post-Test Items

Item	Response Options
Family-centered treatment—general questions How much do you feel you already know about the [NAME] model? How much do you feel you already know about infant-caregiver attachment?	• A great deal • Some • A little • Nothing at all
Family-centered treatment—specific questions	
Nurturing Parenting: The most critical aspect of nurturing is empathy. Nurturing Parenting: Parents cannot nurture their children if they do not nurture themselves.	• Strongly agree • Agree • Neutral • Disagree • Strongly disagree
Promoting First Relationships: Which of the following is NOT part of the concept of a "secure base"?	• A caregiver who is consistently sensitive and responsive • A caregiver who supports the need for exploration • A caregiver who maintains consistent physical contact with her/his child • A caregiver who maintains consistent love, attention, and protection
Promoting First Relationships: The four Promoting First Relationships Consultation Strategies are join with caregivers; engage in reflective observation; give verbal feedback, and:	• Ask reflective questions • Provide positive guidance • Assist with describing consequences • Advise in setting schedules
Partners in Parenting Education: It is important for caregivers to be able to correctly define emotion in infant faces.	• Strongly agree • Agree • Neutral • Disagree • Strongly disagree
Partners in Parenting Education: Helping caregivers feel more confident starts with helping caregivers understand their infants' cues.	• Strongly agree • Agree • Neutral • Disagree • Strongly disagree

Table A.10—Continued

Item	Response Options
Evidence-Based Practice Attitude Scale	
Please circle the response below each item that indicates the extent to which you agree with the statement.	
I like to use new types of therapy/interventions to help my clients.	
I am willing to try new types of therapy/interventions even if I have to follow a treatment manual.	
I know better than academic researchers how to care for my clients.	• Not at all
I am willing to use new and different types of therapy/interventions developed by researchers.	• To a slight extent • To a moderate extent • To a great extent
Research-based treatments/interventions are not clinically useful.	• To a very great extent.
Clinical experience is more important than using manualized therapy/interventions.	
I would not use manualized therapy/interventions.	
I would try a new therapy/intervention even if it were very different from what I am used to doing.	
If you received training in a therapy or intervention that was new to you, how likely would you be to adopt it if:	
It was intuitively appealing?	
It "made sense" to you?	
It was required by your supervisor?	• Not at all
It was required by your agency?	• To a slight extent • To a moderate extent • To a great extent
It was required by the state?	• To a very great extent
It was being used by colleagues who were happy with it?	
You felt you had enough training to use it correctly?	

Nurturing Parenting Training

The goal of the training was to provide an introduction to the principles of the Nurturing Parenting model, and to assist providers in incorporating these principles into the services they provide. The Nurturing Parenting program was originally developed to prevent and/or treat child abuse and neglect. The program addresses several components of the parent-child relationship, including child development, emotional connections, discipline, communication, and coping with stress. Nineteen individuals participated in the training; seven completed training evaluation surveys.

Individuals participating in the training represented a range of educational and professional backgrounds. Approximately one-half of the participants identified their specialty as social work or clinical social work, the remainder identifying their specialty as "other." The majority of participants indicated some specialty training beyond a bachelor's degree, including master's degree, master's of social work, or licensure in social work. All participants reported experience in administering individual therapy for children, and nearly all reported experience with individual therapy for parents and relationship-based interventions. Most participants reported experience working with infants and preschool children.

On the pre-training survey, participants were asked to complete the Evidence-Based Practice Attitudes Scale (Aarons, 2004), described above. Participants indicated that they would incorporate new therapies in moderate to great extents if the new therapy were required (m=3.14) or appealing (m=3.92). Participants also expressed moderate to great openness to new therapies (m=3.82), and only slight resistance to the use of manualized/research-based interventions (m=2.18).

Perceived knowledge about nurturing parenting and infant-caregiver attachment appeared to increase (Table A.11) as indicated by an increase in score on the measure. However, we did not conduct statistical tests because of the small sample size.

Training participants also appeared to change their knowledge of the model in the expected direction (Table A.12). For these items, an increase in score represents improvement on the measure. However, we did not conduct statistical tests because of the small sample size.

After the training, participants reported on average that they were "very confident" that they could deliver treatment consistent with the Nurturing Parenting model. They also reported agreement to strong agreement that the workshop was worthwhile, that they gained valuable knowledge about providing treatment to these at-risk families, and that they learned things they didn't know about treating depressed caregivers and helping families with children affected by developmental delays.

Promoting First Relationships Training

The goal of the training was to provide participants with information about the Promoting First Relationships model, and to assist them with using these principles in their interactions with families. Promoting First Relationships emphasizes the importance of attachment between infants/toddlers and their parents/caregivers with a focus on the potentially negative impacts of poverty, family stress, special needs, and behavioral problems on the parent-child relationship. A total of 152 participants completed training assessment surveys.

Individuals participating in the training represented a range of educational and professional backgrounds. About a quarter of participants reported that their professional degree was a bachelor's degree, more than half reported a master's degree, and other participants reported specialty training (e.g., master's of social work, registered nurses, or doctorate degrees) or identified their degree/certification as "other." Approximately 7 percent of attendees were early intervention service coordinators, and an additional 11 percent were social workers or clinical social workers. Approximately 3 percent were nurses. Due to increased attendance by particular specialties, we included additional categories in the survey for the three training sessions in 2011. Of the 89 participants who completed those sessions, approximately 30 percent were

Table A.11
Knowledge of Nurturing Parenting and Attachment

Item	Pre	Post
Knowledge about the Nurturing Parenting model	3.29	4.29
Knowledge about infant-caregiver attachment	4.00	4.29

NOTE: 1=nothing at all, 4=a great deal.

Table A.12
Knowledge of Nurturing Parenting Model

Belief	Pre	Post
The most critical aspect of nurturing is empathy	4.00	4.57
Parents cannot nurture their children if they do not nurture themselves	4.71	5.00

NOTE: 1=strongly disagree, 5=strongly agree.

speech/language pathologists, 24 percent occupational therapists, 17 percent developmentalists, 10 percent physical therapists, and 6 percent behavioral health therapists. The remaining attendees identified their specialty as "other."

With respect to clinical experience, more than 75 percent of the participants reported experience in administering individual therapy for children and just under half reported experience with group therapy for children. For parent-focused therapy, approximately one quarter of the participants reported experience with individual therapy for parents and 11 percent reported experience with group therapy for parents. More than half of the participants had experience administering relationship-based interventions. Overall, more than 85 percent of participants reported experience working with infants or toddlers, and more than 75 percent reported previous experience working with preschool children.

On the Evidence-Based Practice Attitudes Scale administered before training began, participants indicated that they would incorporate new therapies to a moderate to great extent if the new therapy were required (m=3.73, SD=.99) or appealing (m=3.78, SD=.78). Participants also expressed moderate to great openness to new therapies (m=3.55, SD=.58), and only slight resistance to the use of manualized/research-based interventions (m=2.26, SD=.78).

Perceived knowledge about the Promoting First Relationships model and infant-caregiver attachment showed significant improvement from pre- to post-training (Table A.13). For these items, an increase in score represents improvement on the measure.

Training participants also completed a brief two-item quiz on the Promoting First Relationships model before and after the training. Based on chi-square difference tests, participants demonstrated significant improvement in the percentage correct for the questions pertaining to a "secure base" ($\chi^2[1]=8.19$, p<.01) and Promoting First Relationships Consultation Strategies ($\chi^2[1]=5.75$, p<.05). Of the participants who completed the quiz before and after training, approximately 25 percent of participants improved performance on the quiz. In contrast, fewer than 7 percent declined in performance on one or more items (Table A.14).

Table A.13
Knowledge of Promoting First Relationships and Attachment

Item	Pre	Post	Significance Level
Knowledge about the Promoting First Relationships model	3.05	4.49	<.001
Knowledge about infant-caregiver attachment	3.98	4.54	<.001

NOTE: 1=nothing at all, 4=a great deal.

Table A.14
Knowledge of Promoting First Relationships Model

Item (Correct Answer Is in Parentheses)	Pre	Post	Significance Level
Which of the following is NOT part of the concept of a "secure base?" (A caregiver who maintains consistent physical contact with her/his child)	66%	85%	<.01
The four Promoting First Relationships Consultation Strategies are: join with caregivers; engage in reflective observation; give verbal feedback, and (ask reflective questions)	40%	70%	<.05

NOTE: Chi-square tests were conducted to test significant difference between pre- and post-training performance.

After the training, participants reported on average that they were "very confident" that they could deliver treatment consistent with the Promoting First Relationships model. They also reported that the workshop was worthwhile, that they gained valuable knowledge about providing treatment to at-risk families, and that they learned things they didn't know about treating depressed caregivers and helping families with children affected by developmental delays.

Partners in Parenting Education

The goal of the training was to introduce participants to the concepts of Partners in Parenting Education, and to assist them in integrating these principles into their work with families. Partners in Parenting Education aims to promote healthy infant-parent relationships with a focus on developing and maintaining secure attachments between children and caregivers. A total of 25 training participants completed evaluation surveys.

Individuals participating in the training represented a wide range of professional education and specialty. Approximately 20 percent of attendees were social workers or clinical social workers, and nearly 10 percent were early intervention service coordinators. The remaining participants represented a broad diversity of occupations, including psychologist, speech therapist, physical therapist, and manager. Around 33 percent of participants reported a bachelor's degree, approximately 40 percent reported a master's degree, and the remaining participants reported specialty training (e.g., a master's of social work) or identified their degree/certification as "other." Approximately three quarters of the participants reported experience in administering individual therapy for children, and approximately half reported experience with individual therapy for parents. Nearly 70 percent indicated that they had previous experience administering relationship-based interventions. Furthermore, more than 90 percent of participants reported experience working with infants and preschool children.

As with the other relationship-based intervention trainings, participants were asked to complete the Evidence-Based Practice Attitudes Scale (Aarons, 2004) before training began to assess attitudes toward using evidence-based therapies and interventions. Participants indicated that they would incorporate new therapies to a moderate to great extent if the new therapy were required (m=3.60) or appealing (m=4.12). Participants also expressed moderate to great openness to new therapies (m=3.81), and only slight resistance to the use of manualized/research-based interventions (m=2.13).

Perceived knowledge about the Partners in Parenting Education model and infant-caregiver attachment showed improvement from pre- to post-training (Table A.15). For these items, an increase in score represents improvement on the measure.

Training participants did not demonstrate substantial changes in their knowledge of the Partners in Parenting Education, but this is likely due to their strong endorsement of the Partners in Parenting Education principles prior to the training (Table A.16).

Table A.15
Knowledge of Partners in Parenting Education and Attachment

Item	Pre	Post	Significance Level
Knowledge about the Partners in Parenting Education model	2.92	4.37	<.01
Knowledge about infant-caregiver attachment	4.20	4.56	<.05

NOTE: 1=nothing at all, 4=a great deal.

Table A.16
Knowledge of Partners in Parenting Education Model

Belief	Pre	Post	Significance Level
It is important for caregivers to be able to correctly define emotion in infant faces.	4.36	4.84	n.s.
Helping caregivers feel more confident starts with helping caregivers understand their infant's cues.	4.48	4.80	n.s.

NOTE: 1=strongly disagree, 5=strongly agree; n.s.=non-significant.

After the training, participants reported on average that they were "very confident" that they could deliver treatment consistent with the Partners in Parenting Education model. They also reported that the workshop was a worthwhile event, that they gained valuable knowledge about providing treatment to at risk families, and that they learned things they didn't know about treating depressed caregivers and helping families with children affected by developmental delays.

Training Evaluation Summary

More than 300 early intervention and behavioral health providers participated in trainings on the initiative, the referral processes, infant mental health, relationship-based care, and specific relationship-based intervention models. Overall, training participants demonstrated significant improvement in knowledge about the screening and referral processes, the critical effects of maternal depression on the early development of the brain, infant-caregiver attachment, and relationship-based care.

Data Collection Tools

In this appendix, we offer reproductions of our data collection tools. Figures B.1–B.7 include the screening and assessment packet; behavioral health provider and early intervention focus group protocols; service coordinator focus group protocol; family interview discussion guide; screening/assessment tracking form; and referral tracking form.

Figure B.1
Screening and Assessment Packet

Helping
Families
Raise
Healthy
Children

Caregiver Name	EI Number	Project ID

Baseline	6 month	12 month	18 month	24 month

Caregiver Screening/Assessment Packet

Please note that:

- Participation is voluntary – **you do not have to complete this packet.**
- All information you provide will be kept **confidential.**
- Screening will help the Alliance understand your family's needs. Some of the screening questions may ask about sensitive or emotional issues. **You are still eligible to receive services if you decline to be screened.**
- The information you provide may be used in a project that the Alliance is doing to learn how to improve the services they provide. RAND Corporation, a non-profit research organization here in Pittsburgh, will be analyzing the data that the Alliance collects. The data sent to RAND will be marked with an identification number only. Your name or your child's name will not be shared with RAND.
- **You may decline to have your information be a part of this project.** You can fill out the screening packet to help the Alliance understand your family's needs, but can require that it not be a part of the data that is shared with RAND.
- Screening is provided at no cost to families.
- **All information is confidential.** The information you provide may be used to inform ongoing quality improvement efforts at the Alliance.
- You will have the opportunity to describe your child and discuss any concerns you may have.

Please tell us your preference below:
I will fill out the screening packet, and you may share de-identified information from this packet with RAND.

I will fill out the screening packet, but you <u>may not</u> share de-identified information from this packet with RAND.

Figure B.1—Continued

Helping
Families
Raise
Healthy
Children

Service Coordinator: _____ **Screening Date:** _____

Over the past two weeks, have you been bothered by any of the following problems?

Little interest or pleasure in doing things.   **YES**   **NO**

Feeling down, depressed, or hopeless.   **YES**   **NO**

Figure B.1—Continued

Helping
Families
Raise
Healthy
Children

Service Coordinator: _____ **Screening Date:** _____

Based on what you just told me, I want to ask about some things that might have been bothering you recently. Your answers will help me figure out how best to support you and your family.

Over the last weeks, how often have you been bothered by any of the following problems?

	Not at all	Several days	More than half the days	Nearly every day
1. Little interest or pleasure in doing things	0	1	2	3
2. Feeling down, depressed, or hopeless	0	1	2	3
3. Trouble falling asleep or staying asleep, or sleeping too much	0	1	2	3
4. Feeling tired or having little energy	0	1	2	3
5. Poor appetite or overeating	0	1	2	3
6. Feeling bad about yourself or that you are a failure or have let yourself or your family down	0	1	2	3
7. Trouble concentrating on things, such as reading the newspaper or watching television	0	1	2	3
8. Moving or speaking so slowly that other people could have noticed. Or the opposite – being so fidgety or restless that you have been moving around a lot more than usual	0	1	2	3
9. Thoughts that you would be better off dead, or of hurting yourself	0	1	2	3

Add columns

Total point score:

_____

Figure B.1—Continued

Service Coordinator: _____   **Screening Date:** _____

We would also like to ask you a few questions about your physical health.

1. Would you say that in general your health is…?

Excellent	1
Very Good	2
Good	3
Fair	4
Poor	5

2. During the past 30 days, for about how many days have you felt you did not get enough rest or sleep?

    _____

3. In general, how healthy is your overall diet? Would you say…?

Excellent	1
Very Good	2
Good	3
Fair	4
Poor	5

4. During the past month, did you participate in any physical activities or exercises such as running, calisthenics, golf, gardening, or walking for exercise?

Yes	1
No	2

5. What kind of place do you USUALLY go to when you need routine or preventive care, such as a physical examination or check-up?

Doesn't get preventive care anywhere	1
Clinic or health center	2
Doctor's office or HMO	3
Hospital emergency room	4
Hospital outpatient department	5
Some other place	6
Doesn't go to one place most often	7

Figure B.1—Continued

6.   During the past 6 months, how many times have you gone to a hospital emergency room about your own health (This includes emergency room visits that resulted in a hospital admission.)?

           _____

7.   Are you currently in a relationship that is not safe?

           Yes   1
           No   2

8.   **[IF 7=YES]** Would you like to speak to someone about this for available resources?

           Yes   1
           No   2

9.   During the past 6 months, how many times has your child gone to a hospital emergency room about (his/her) health (This includes emergency room visits that resulted in a hospital admission.)?

           _____   ☐   Check if for NICU or other chronic health issue

10.   Does the child have a physician that he/she sees regularly?

           Yes   1
           No   2

11.   Based on the American Academy of Pediatric Standards, are the child's immunizations up-to-date?

           Yes   1
            No   2

Figure B.1—Continued

Service Coordinator: _____   **Screening Date:** _____

Earlier you said that some things were bothering you. We have some more questions about how you are feeling. Read the statements below.

Mark **SA** if you <u>strongly agree</u> with the statement
Mark **A** if you <u>agree</u> with the statement
Mark **NS** if you are <u>not sure</u>
Mark **D** if you <u>disagree</u> with the statement
Mark **SD** if you <u>strongly disagree</u> with the statement

	SA (5)	A (4)	NS (3)	D (2)	SD (1)
1. I often have the feeling that I cannot handle things very well.	O	O	O	O	O
2. I find myself giving up more of my life to meet my children's needs than I ever expected.	O	O	O	O	O
3. I feel trapped by my responsibilities as a parent.	O	O	O	O	O
4. Since having this child, I have been unable to do new and different things.	O	O	O	O	O
5. Since having a child, I feel that I am almost never able to do things that I like to do.	O	O	O	O	O
6. I am unhappy with the last purchase of clothing I made for myself.	O	O	O	O	O
7. There are quite a few things that bother me about my life.	O	O	O	O	O
8. Having a child has caused more problems than I expected in my relationship with my spouse (male/female friend).	O	O	O	O	O
9. I feel alone and without friends.	O	O	O	O	O
10. When I go to a party, I usually expect not to enjoy myself.	O	O	O	O	O
11. I am not as interested in people as I used to be.	O	O	O	O	O
12. I don't enjoy things as I used to.	O	O	O	O	O
13. My child rarely does things for me that make me feel good.	O	O	O	O	O
14. Most times I feel that my child does not like me and does not want to be close to me.	O	O	O	O	O
15. My child smiles at me much less than I expected.	O	O	O	O	O
16. When I do things for my child, I get the feeling that my efforts are not appreciated very much.	O	O	O	O	O
17. When playing, my child doesn't often giggle or laugh.	O	O	O	O	O
18. My child doesn't seem to learn as quickly as most children.	O	O	O	O	O
19. My child doesn't seem to smile as much as most children.	O	O	O	O	O
20. My child is not able to do as much as I expected.	O	O	O	O	O
21. It takes a long time and it is very hard for my child to get used to new things.	O	O	O	O	O

Figure B.1—Continued

For the next statement, choose your response from the choices "1" to "5" below.

22. I feel that I am: 1 2 3 4 5
    1. not very good at being a parent
    2. a person who has some trouble being a parent
    3. an average parent
    4. a better than average parent
    5. a very good parent

	SA (5)	A (4)	NS (3)	D (2)	SD (1)
23. I expected to have closer and warmer feelings for my child than I do and this bothers me.	O	O	O	O	O
24. Sometimes my child does things that bother me just to be mean.	O	O	O	O	O
25. My child seems to cry or fuss more often than most children.	O	O	O	O	O
26. My child generally wakes up in a bad mood.	O	O	O	O	O
27. I feel that my child is very moody and easily upset.	O	O	O	O	O
28. My child does a few things which bother me a great deal.	O	O	O	O	O
29. My child reacts very strongly when something happens that my child doesn't like.	O	O	O	O	O
30. My child gets upset easily over the smallest thing.	O	O	O	O	O
31. My child's sleeping or eating schedule was much harder to establish than expected.	O	O	O	O	O

For the next statement, choose your response from the choices "1" to "5" below.

32. I have found that getting my child to do something or stop doing something is: 1 2 3 4 5
    1. much harder than I expected
    2. somewhat harder than I expected
    3. about as hard as I expected
    4. somewhat easier than I expected
    5. much easier than I expected

For the next statement, choose your response from the choices "10+" to "1-3."

33. Think carefully and count the number of things which your child does that bother you. For example: dawdles, refuses to listen, overactive, cries, interrupts, fights, whines, etc.   10+ 8-9 6-7 4-5 1-3

	SA (5)	A (4)	NS (3)	D (2)	SD (1)
34. There are some things my child does that really bother me a lot.	O	O	O	O	O
35. My child turned out to be more of a problem than I had expected.	O	O	O	O	O
36. My child makes more demands on me than most children.	O	O	O	O	O

Figure B.2
Behavioral Health Provider Focus Group Protocol

Helping Families Raise Healthy Children
Stakeholder Discussion Outline
Behavioral Health Providers

I.   Referrals to Behavioral Health Resulting from HFRHC

- Referral method
- In general, how is the referral process going?
- Appropriateness of referrals
- Caregiver follow-through on appointments
- How does caregiver follow-through compare to clients who are referred from other sources?

II. Mobile Therapy

- Initial reactions to providing mobile therapy for families referred from HFRHC
- How are things going now that the process has been in place for a while?
- Differences in caregiver uptake
- Successes related to providing mobile therapy
- Challenges related to providing mobile therapy
- Recommendations to other agencies/providers considering mobile therapy

III. Training on Family Centered Interventions

- Quality of training
- Quantity of training
- Usefulness of training for ongoing work
- Would you recommend the training for other providers
- What continuing training would be helpful?

IV. Use of Family Centered Interventions

- Are you using any of the family-centered techniques?
- Implementation of techniques learned (i.e. how has it changed your approach to working with families?)
- Successes related to using the approach with families
- Challenges related to using the approach with families
- Recommendations for other BH providers regarding use of approach in their work with families

Figure B.2—Continued

V.   Communication/Collaboration

- Changes in quantity or quality of communications with the Alliance and/or Early Intervention providers
- Changes in amount/type of collaboration among various providers since the initiative has been in place
- Successes related to communicating/collaborating with the Alliance and/or Early Intervention providers
- Challenges related to communication/collaboration among various providers
- Recommendations to enhance communication/collaboration among various providers

VI.   Learning Collaborative

- Level of participation in Learning Collaborative activities
- Usefulness of Learning Collaborative for ongoing work
- Recommendations for improving the Learning Collaborative
- Would you recommend the Learning Collaborative for other providers

Figure B.3
Early Intervention Focus Group Protocol

Helping Families Raise Healthy Children
Stakeholder Discussion Outline
Early Intervention Providers

I. Referrals to EI involving Caregiver Depression

- Process for referrals that also involve caregiver depression
- In general, how is the process going?
- Appropriateness of referrals involving caregiver depression
- Caregiver follow-through on appointments
- How does caregiver follow-through compare to clients who are not affected by depression?

II. Providing Services Related to Caregiver Depression

- Initial reactions to providing services related to caregiver depression
- How are things going now that the process has been in place for a while?
- Differences in how families receive services
- Successes related to providing these services
- Challenges related to providing these services
- Recommendations to other agencies/providers considering providing these services within the early intervention system

III. Training on Family Centered Interventions

- Quality of training
- Quantity of training
- Usefulness of training for ongoing work
- Would you recommend the training for other providers
- What continuing training would be helpful?

IV. Use of Family Centered Interventions

- Are you using any of the family-centered techniques?
- Implementation of techniques learned (i.e. how has it changed your approach to working with families?)
- Successes related to using the approach with families
- Challenges related to using the approach with families
- Recommendations for other EI providers regarding use of approach in their work with families

Figure B.3—Continued

V. Ongoing Communication/Collaboration

- Changes in quantity or quality of communications with the Alliance and/or Behavioral Health providers
- Changes in amount/type of collaboration among various providers since the initiative has been in place
- Successes related to communicating/collaborating with the Alliance and/or Behavioral Health providers
- Challenges related to communication/collaboration with the Alliance and/or Behavioral Health providers
- Recommendations to enhance communication/collaboration among various providers

VI. Learning Collaborative

- Level of participation in Learning Collaborative activities
- Usefulness of Learning Collaborative for ongoing work
- Recommendations for improving the Learning Collaborative
- Would you recommend the Learning Collaborative for other providers

Figure B.4
Service Coordinator Focus Group Protocol

Helping Families Raise Healthy Children
Stakeholder Discussion Outline
Alliance Service Coordinators

I. Screening
  - Initial reaction to new screening protocol for caregivers
  - Successes related to screening
  - Challenges related to screening
  - Recommendations for systematic screening by Service Coordinators
  - Additional training/support needed for screening

II. Assessments
  - Use of information from assessments (PSI, caregiver and child health)
  - Challenges related to completing assessments
  - Recommendations for completing assessments
  - Additional training/support needed for assessments

III. Referrals
  - Use of Alliance Mental Health Specialists as a resource?
  - Do you feel equipped to respond to positive screens or caregiver request for referrals now?
  - Additional training/support/resources needed for referral process
  - Family reactions to referrals for caregiver depression
  - Family feedback on complete/incomplete referrals for caregiver depression
  - Recommendations to enhance referral process and uptake of services

IV. Ongoing Communication/Collaboration
  - Changes in quantity or quality of communications with Early Intervention, Behavioral Health and other community providers
  - Changes in amount/type of collaboration among various providers since the initiative has been in place
  - Successes related to communicating/collaborating with Early Intervention, Behavioral Health and other community providers
  - Challenges related to communication/collaboration with Early Intervention, Behavioral Health and other community providers
  - Recommendations to enhance communication/collaboration among various providers

V. Relationship-Based Interventions
  - Participation in training on relationship-based interventions
  - Usefulness of training for ongoing work
  - Implementation of techniques learned (i.e. how has it changed your approach to working with families?)
  - Successes related to using the approach with families
  - Challenges related to using the approach with families
  - Additional support/training needed to use the approach

Figure B.5
Service Coordinator Focus Group Protocol

Helping Families Raise Healthy Children

Discussion Outline for Family/Caregiver Interviews

In the past year, we've been working with the Alliance on an ongoing project to help identify stress and depression among parents and caregivers of children at risk for developmental delays. We're currently talking to families to learn more about their experiences with this process and really appreciate your willingness to talk to us about your personal experience. We want to know both about the things that went well and the things that we could make better. We think of this conversation as a partnership to help us improve this process for families. I will have some more specific questions for you throughout our conversation, but I thought it would be great if you could first tell me a little bit about your experience. Did you talk to your Service Coordinator from the Alliance, [*insert name*] about parental stress or depression? What happened after that?

I. Screening
- How did you feel about talking to your service coordinator about parental stress or depression?
  - Were you comfortable answering his/her questions?
  - Did you have any concerens about the process?
- Is there anything you would have changed about the process?
- Is there anything we could have done to make the conversation with your service coordinator a little easier?
- Has your service coordinator checked in with you about how you're feeling since your first conversation about this? How often would you like your service coordinator to ask you about parental stress and depression?
- Have you ever been asked about parental stress or depression in another setting, for example, by your child's pediatrician or your OB?
- Do you have anything else you'd like to say about the process of talking to your service coordinator about parental stress or depression?

II. Referrals
- Did your Alliance Service Coordinator offer any help or connect you to any resources or services to assist with parental stress or depression (e.g., in-home counseling, referral to a family support center)? *[interviewer will have a list of resources and definitions for reference if needed]*
- Were you able to follow up to receive any help based on those recommendations?
- Was it hard or easy to get connected with the help you needed (e.g. scheduling an appointment)? *Probe for further information about response.*
- Do you have any suggestions for improving the process of connecting families to services for parental stress and depression?
- Do you have anything else you'd like to say about the process of getting connected to help for parental stress or depression?

Figure B.5—Continued

III. Services
[Interviewer will be prepared with a description of these services/resources and definitions in case the family member is uncertain about what they are receiving. Due to privacy issues, it's unlikely that we'll be able to identify services the family is receiving in advance.]

- What kinds of help have you received (e.g., counseling, relationship-based therapist)?
- How long did you receive the services?
- Are you still receiving services? If not, why did you stop receiving services?
- What did you like about the services you received? What didn't you like?
- Did the services focus on your relationship with your child(ren)?
- What was your relationship with your child(ren) like before you started receiving services? What was it like afterward? Did your relationship change at all?
- Did you feel like the services were helpful?
- How could we make services for parental stress and depression better?
- *Only for those receiving mental health services:* Has your experience changed the way you think about mental health services?
- Do you have anything else you'd like to say about the services you received for parental stress or depression?

In general, if you had the opportunity to speak with another parent or caregiver, what would you tell them about your experience?

Would you recommend that other agencies ask parents and caregivers about parental stress or depression? [If yes, ask them to identify which agencies or types of services.]

If a family member reveals an ongoing problem during the interview, ask if it's ok to discuss with their service coordinator.

Figure B.6
Screening/Assessment Tracking Form

 Helping
Families
Raise
Healthy
Children

Screening/Assessment Tracking Form
Project ID: _____

Family Information

Child Name: _____

Child Birth Date: _____

Child Sex: _____ Ethnicity: _____

Caregiver Name: _____

Relationship to Child: _____ Caregiver Sex: _____

****

Referral Information

Referral Source (AFIT): _____

Depression Only (Project): _____

Date of Referral: _____

****

Alliance Information

Service Coordinator: _____

☐   New Alliance Family
   o   IFSP
   o   Tracking
   o   Tracking with depression as only risk factor

☐   Existing Alliance Family
   o   IFSP
   o   Tracking
   o   Tracking with depression as only risk factor

****

Screening Information

Screen Date: _____

Screen Result: _____

Figure B.6—Continued

Screening Tracking Information

	Date	Event (Initial home visit, 3-, 6-, 9-month contact, other)	Completed (Yes, No, Refused)	Positive (Yes, No)	Score
Baseline Screen (PHQ-2)					
Baseline Screen (PHQ-9)					
6-Month Screen (PHQ-2)					
6-Month Screen (PHQ-9)					
12-Month Screen (PHQ-2)					
12-Month Screen (PHQ-9)					
18-Month Screen (PHQ-2)					
18-Month Screen (PHQ-9)					
24-Month Screen (PHQ-2)					
24-Month Screen (PHQ-9)					

Comments/reason screens were not offered or declined:

_____

_____

_____

_____

_____

Figure B.6—Continued

Assessment Tracking Information

	Date	Event (Initial home visit, 3-, 6-, 9-month contact, other)	Completed (Yes, No, Refused)	PSI-SF Score
Baseline Assessment				
6-Month Follow-Up Assessment				
12-Month Follow-Up Assessment				
18-Month Follow-Up Assessment				
24-Month Follow-Up Assessment				

Comments/reason assessments were not offered or declined:

_____

_____

_____

_____

_____

Figure B.7
Referral Tracking Form

 Helping
Families
Raise
Healthy
Children

Referral Tracking Form

Proiect ID:

Caregiver Information

Caregiver Name:

_____

Caregiver Birth Date: _____

Caregiver Contact Information:_____

_____

_____

Does this caregiver have Medical Assistance?

Yes   ☐   MA ID #:   _____

No   ☐

Does this caregiver have private insurance?

Yes   ☐   Specify: _____

No   ☐

Comment:_____

Child Information

Child Name:

_____

Child Birth Date: _____

Figure B.7—Continued

Helping
Families
Raise
Healthy
Children

Caregiver Needs

To help tailor services, determine if the caregiver has any of the following (check all that apply):

Alcohol use/abuse or past history	☐
Drug use/abuse or past history	☐
Transportation needs	☐
Domestic violence	☐
Diagnosed mental health disorder (e.g. bipolar disorder)	☐
Currently pregnant or has had a baby within 6 months	☐
Other needs	☐
Specify: _____	

Is the caregiver *currently* receiving behavioral health services?

Yes ☐   From whom: _____
No ☐

If yes, would caregiver like a re-referral to this agency/individual?

Yes ☐
No ☐   Why not: _____

Has the caregiver *ever* received behavioral health services?

Yes ☐   From whom: _____
No ☐

If yes, would caregiver like a re-referral to this agency/individual?

Yes ☐
No ☐   Why not: _____

Currently, would the caregiver like a referral to behavioral health services or other supports?

Yes ☐
No ☐   Why not: _____

Figure B.7—Continued

Helping
Families
Raise
Healthy
Children

Referral Tracking Information

Date	Referred To	Referral Type	Agency Name	Contacted Infant Mental Health Specialist about Referral (Y/N)	Outcome of Referral

Referred To

BH= Behavioral health provider
EI= Early Intervention provider
CC CM= Community Care care manager
MCO CM= Managed Care Organization care manager
OBH= Allegheny County Office of Behavioral Health
RES= Re:solve Crisis Network
FSC= Family Support Center
EHS= Early Head Start
HS= Healthy Start
OCBS= Other Community-Based Services
HFRHC= Infant Mental Health Service Coordination
CYF= Children, Youth and Families

Referral Type

1= In-home mobile therapy
2= Family-focused therapy
3= Outpatient therapy
4= Relationship-based intervention through The Alliance
5= Community-based services (Early Head Start, parenting classes, family support centers, etc.)
6= Crisis intervention
7= Other
8= Family-based therapy

Data Collection Tools   149

Outcome Measure Linkages

Figure C.1 details the linkages between the process and individual-level outcome measures.

Figure C.1
Process and Individual Outcome Measures

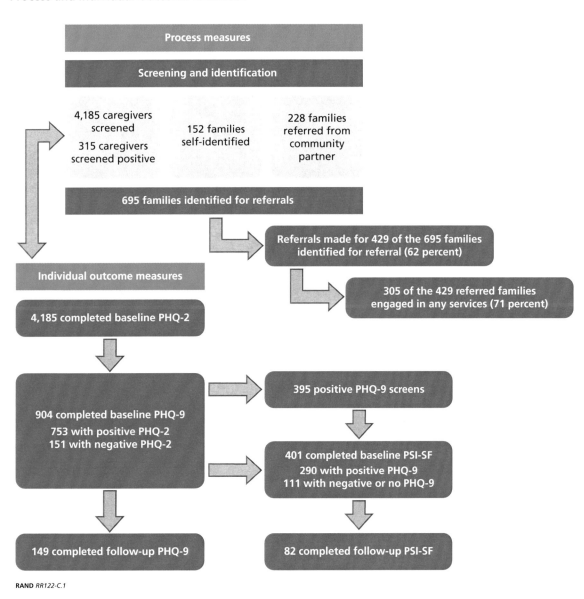

RAND *RR122-C.1*

Reference Studies

Tables D.1–D.3 detail the reference studies used for the screening, referral, and engagement in treatment rate comparisons.

Table D.1
References for Screening Rates from Maternal Depression Literature

Reference	Screening Rate (Base N)	Sample/Respondents	Setting/Study Type	Type of Screening/Notes
Armstrong and Small (2007)	46% (N = 257)	Mothers screened at 4 weeks, 4 months, and 8 months	Descriptive, chart review of rural community pediatric primary care (PPC) clinics	Screening rates varied from 50% at 1 month to 38% at 8 months (total reflects screening rate of all intended screenings). Of the 257 women for whom records were available, 201 were screened at least once. Only 15.5% of participants were screened at all three times.
Garcia, LaCaze, and Ratanasen (2011)	50% (N = 50)	Mothers screened within first six months post birth	Well-child visit at general pediatric clinic	Part of pilot project implementing postpartum depression screening
Gordon et al. (2006)	67% (N not reported)	Perinatal and antenatal depression	Academic medical center OB/GYN	Evaluation of development/implementation of department-based universal perinatal/antenatal depression screening
Heneghan, Morton, and DeLeone (2007)	77% (N = 662)	Maternal depression unspecified	Pediatric providers in community practices	Cross-sectional survey of American Academy of Pediatrics members (45% urban, 65% suburban)
LaRocco-Cockburn et al. (2003)	41% (N = 282)	Adult women (caregiver status not specified)	OB/GYN (49% private practice)	Responded to "often or always screen" for depression
Olson et al. (2002)	8% (N = 508)	Mothers (age of child not specified)	Pediatricians at PPC (56% suburban, 36% urban)	Responded "yes" to "routinely asked about depressive symptoms"
OMAP (2008)	34% (Total N not reported)	Postpartum depression	Chart review on Pennsylvania HealthChoices members	Data are collected via chart review on a sample of participating Medicaid physical health practices across Pennsylvania.
OMAP (2009)	51% (Total N not reported)	Postpartum depression	Chart review on Pennsylvania HealthChoices members	Data are collected via chart review on a sample of participating Medicaid physical health practices across Pennsylvania.
OMAP (2009)	65% (Total N not reported)	Prenatal depression	Chart review on Pennsylvania HealthChoices members	Data are collected via chart review on a sample of participating Medicaid physical health practices across Pennsylvania.
OMAP (2008)	51% (Total N not reported)	Prenatal depression	Chart review on Pennsylvania HealthChoices members	Data are collected via chart review on a sample of participating Medicaid physical health practices across Pennsylvania.
Seehusen et al. (2005)	70% of N = 298	Postpartum depression (age of child not specified)	Family medicine PPC postpartum visits	Survey of Washington Academy of Family Physicians members (83% group practice)
Seehusen et al. (2005)	46% of N = 298	Postpartum depression (age of child not specified)	Family medicine PPC well-child visits	Survey of Washington Academy of Family Physicians members (83% group practice)

Table D.1—Continued

Reference	Screening Rate (Base N)	Sample/Respondents	Setting/Study Type	Type of Screening/ Notes
Segre et al. (2011)	64% of N = 2,694	Perinatal depression	Maternal and child health agencies	Train-the-Trainer Program; Only 16 out of 32 agencies involved in the study provided data. Screening rate is aggregated across the 16 maternal and child health agencies
Thoppil et al. (2005)	75% of N = 109	Perinatal depression, women >32 weeks gestation	Chart review at outpatient obstetrics clinic	Evaluation of intervention for screening for perinatal depression

NOTE: Mean across references = 53%, median = 51%, minimum = 8%, maximum = 77%. All references include low-income samples.

Table D.2
References for Referral Rates from Maternal Depression Literature

Reference	Referral Rate (Base N)	Sample	Setting/Study Type	Type of Referral/Notes
Yonkers et al. (2009)	9% (N = 367)	Pregnant and postpartum women	Obstetrical care at publicly funded health care clinics	Pre-Healthy Start; all women who requested or required a treatment referral were given the names and numbers of at least two providers. In addition, the New Haven Healthy Start program offered weekly drop-in services that provided behavioral services, pharmacological services, or both to participants. Participants were contacted again after one, three, and six months, and additional referrals were given, if necessary.
Yonkers et al. (2009)	2% (N = 969)	Pregnant and postpartum women	Obstetrical care at publicly funded health care clinics	Post-Healthy Start; same as above.
Chaudron et al. (2004).	50% (N=16)	Postpartum depression in first year after birth	Well-child visits at pediatric clinics in large academic setting	Social work referrals
OMAP (2009)	52% (N not reported)	Prenatal depression	Chart review on HealthChoices members	Data are collected via chart review on a sample of participating Medicaid physical health practices across Pennsylvania.
OMAP (2008)	61% (N not reported)	Prenatal depression	Chart review on HealthChoices members	Data are collected via chart review on a sample of participating Medicaid physical health practices across Pennsylvania.
OMAP (2009)	68% (N not reported)	Postpartum depression	Chart review on HealthChoices members	Data are collected via chart review on a sample of participating Medicaid physical health practices across Pennsylvania.
OMAP (2008)	73% (N not reported)	Postpartum depression	Chart review on HealthChoices members	Data are collected via chart review on a sample of participating Medicaid physical health practices across Pennsylvania.
Sheeder et al. (2009)	100% (N = 413)	Postpartum depression within six months of birth for adolescent mothers	Colorado Adolescent Maternity Program (CAMP) in Community Hospital	If > 22 years old, referred to community mental health agencies. If < 22 years old, evaluated by the clinic social worker or referred for further evaluation. 100% referral due to use of EPIC computer system. If Edinburgh Postnatal Depression Scale score > 10, providers could not close medical record until management plan or referral had been recorded.

NOTE: Mean across references = 51.6%, median = 56.1%, minimum = 1.0%, maximum = 100.0%. All references include low-income samples.

Table D.3
References for Engagement Rates from Maternal Depression Literature

Reference	Engagement Rate		Sample	Setting	Types of Services	Notes
	<1 session (Base N)	Multiple sessions (Base N)				
Miranda et al. (2003)	17% of N = 87	17% of N = 87	Women with current major depression	Screened and referred at Women, Infants and Children (WIC) program	Community mental health care clinician	Engagement defined as participating in one session or more; 25% of the women declined referral. Referred participants were contacted to encourage them to attend the intake appointment for care.
Sit et al. (2009)	16% (N not reported)	Not reported	Postpartum depression (child age not specified)	Healthy Start Program	Mental health or social services	Engagement defined as attending initial appointment; because this is a secondary review of the annual report of Healthy Start of Pittsburgh, base N is not available.
Smith, Shao, et al. (2009)	38% (N = 465)	6% of N = 465	Perinatal and postpartum women	Publicly funded obstetric clinics	Mental health services	All referred as part of study; 38.1% attended at least one mental health visit; 6% remained in treatment during the entire six-month follow-up interval.
Wiggins et al. (2005)	19% (N=184)	Not reported	Postnatal women with infant ten weeks old	Community group services	Community group support	All mothers referred as part of intervention study. Engagement defined as having at least one visit.
Wiggins et al. (2005)	94% (N=184)	Not reported	Postnatal women with infant ten weeks old	Home visits	Home visits	All mothers referred as part of intervention study. Engagement defined as having at least one visit.

NOTE: Mean across references = 36.8%, median = 19.0%, minimum = 16.0%, maximum = 94.0%. Referral rates were not reported in the original reference, unless noted otherwise. All references include low-income samples.

Bibliography

Aarons GA. "Mental health provider attitudes toward adoption of evidence-based practice: The Evidence-Based Practice Attitude Scale (EBPAS)." *Mental Health Services Research,* 2004, 6(2): 61–74.

Abidin RR. *Parenting Stress Index—Third Edition.* Lutz, Fla.: Psychological Assessment Resources, 1995.

Abrams LS, Dornig K, Curran L. "Barriers to service use for postpartum depression symptoms among low-income ethnic minority mothers in the United States." *Qualitative Health Research,* 2009, 19(4): 535–551.

Adams KG, Greiner AC, Corrigan JM, eds. *The 1st Annual Crossing the Quality Chasm Summit: A Focus on Communities.* Conference report, Washington, D.C.: National Academies Press, 2004.

Administration for Children and Families. "Research to practice brief: Depression in the lives of Early Head Start families," Washington, DC: U.S. Department of Health and Human Services, 2006.

Agency for Healthcare Research and Quality. "National healthcare disparities report: Summary," Rockville, Md.: Agency for Healthcare Research and Quality, 2004.

Allegheny County Maternal and Child Health Care Collaborative. *Building a Model Maternal and Child Health Care System in the Pittsburgh Region: A Community-Based Quality Improvement Effort.* Santa Monica, Calif.: RAND Corporation, 2006.

American Congress of Obstetricians and Gynecologists, Committee on Obstetric Practice. "Committee opinion no. 354: Treatment with selective serotonin reuptake inhibitors during pregnancy." *Obstetrics and Gynecology,* 2006, (108): 1601–1603.

Armstrong S, Small R. "Screening for postnatal depression: Not a simple task." *Australian and New Zealand Journal of Public Health,* 2007, 31(1): 57–61.

Arroll B, Goodyear-Smith F, Crengle S, Gunn J, Kerse N, Fishman T, Falloon K, Hatcher S. "Validation of PHQ-2 and PHQ-9 to screen for major depression in the primary care population." *Annals of Family Medicine,* 2010, 8: 348–353.

Barlow J, Coren E. "Parent-training programmes for improving maternal psychosocial health." *Cochrane Database System Review(1),* 2004, CD002020.

Beck CT, "Maternal depression and child behaviour problems: A meta-analysis." *Journal of Advanced Nursing,* 1999, 29(3): 623–629.

Beeber L, Holditch-Davis D, Belyea M, Funk SG, Canuso R. "In-home intervention for depressive symptoms with low-income mothers of infants and toddlers in the United States." Health Care for Women International, 2004, 25: 561–580.

Beeber L, Holditch-Davis D, Perreira K, Schwartz T, Lewis V, Blanchard H, Canuso R, Davis Goldman B. "Short-term in-home intervention reduces depressive symptoms in Early Head Start Latina mothers of infants and toddlers." *Research in Nursing and Health,* 2010, 33(1): 60–76.

Beeghly M, Olson KL, Weinberg MK, Pierre SC, Downey N, Tronick EZ. "Prevalence, stability, and socio-demographic correlates of depressive symptoms in black mothers during the first 18 months postpartum." *Maternal and Child Health Journal,* 2003, 7(3): 157–168.

Beeghly M, Weinberg MK, Olson KL, Kernan H, Riley J, Tronick EZ. "Stability and change in level of maternal depressive symptomatology during the first postpartum year." *Journal of Affective Disorders,* 2002, 71(1–3): 169–180.

Bennett IM, Marcus SC, Palmer SC, Coyne JC. "Pregnancy-related discontinuation of antidepressants and depression care visits among Medicaid recipients." *Psychiatric Services,* 2010, 61(4): 386–391.

Bethell C, Peck C, Schor E. "Assessing health system provision of well-child care: The Promoting Healthy Development Survey." *Pediatrics,* 2001, 107(5): 1084–1094.

Birndorf CA, Madden A, Portera L, Leon AC. "Psychiatric symptoms, functional impairment, and receptivity toward mental health treatment among obstetrical patients." *International Journal of Psychiatry in Medicine,* 2001, 31(4): 355–365.

Bloom B, Cohen RA, Freeman G. "Summary health statistics for US children: National Health Interview Survey, 2008." *Vital and Health Statistics,* 2009, 244: 1.

Bonari L, Pinto N, Ahn A, Einarson A, Steiner M, Koren G. "Perinatal risks of untreated depression during pregnancy." *Canadian Journal of Psychiatry,* 2004, 49(11): 726–735.

Boyd RC, Mogul M, Newman D, Coyne JC. "Screening and referral for postpartum depression among low-income women: A qualitative perspective from community health workers." *Depression Research and Treatment,* 2011, Article ID 320605.

Browne JV, Talmi A. "Family-based intervention to enhance infant-parent relationships in the neonatal intensive care unit." *Journal of Pediatric Psychology,* 2005, 30(8): 667–677.

Bureau of Health Statistics and Research. "2008 Behavioral Health Risks of Pennsylvania Adults." Harrisburg, Pa.: Bureau of Health Statistics and Research, 2009.

Carter FA, Carter JD, Luty SE, Wilson DA, Frampton CM, Joyce PR. "Screening and treatment for depression during pregnancy: A cautionary note." *Australia New Zealand Journal of Psychiatry.* 2005, 39(4): 255–261.

Center on the Developing Child at Harvard University. "Maternal depression can undermine the development of young children: Working Paper No. 8." Cambridge Mass.: Center on the Developing Child at Harvard University, 2009. As of February 12, 2013: http://developingchild.harvard.edu/index.php/resources/reports_and_working_papers/working_papers/wp8/

Centers for Disease Control and Prevention. "Prevalence of self-reported postpartum depressive symptoms—17 states, 2004–2005." *Morbidity and Mortality Weekly Report,* 2008, 57(14): 361–366.

Chapman DP, Wheaton AG, Perry GS, Sturgis SL, Strine TW, Croft JB. "Household demographics and perceived insufficient sleep among US adults." *Journal of Community Health,* 2012, 37(2): 344–349.

Chaudron LH, Szilagyi PG, Kitzman HJ, Wadkins HIM, Conwell Y. "Detection of postpartum depressive symptoms by screening at well-child visits." *Pediatrics,* 2004, 113(3): 551–558.

Children's Defense Fund of Minnesota. *Maternal Depression and Early Childhood.* Zero to Three Research to Policy Project, 2011. As of February 12, 2013: http://www.cdf-mn.org/multimedia-and-news/news-from-cdf-minnesota/2011/maternal-depression-and-early.html

Cicchetti D, Rogosch FA, Toth SL. "The efficacy of toddler-parent psychotherapy for fostering cognitive development in offspring of depressed mothers." *Journal of Abnormal Child Psychology,* 2000, 28: 135–148.

Clark R, Tluczek A, Wenzel A. "Psychotherapy for postpartum depression: A preliminary report." *American Journal of Orthopsychiatry,* 2003, 73: 441–454.

Commonwealth of Pennsylvania. "Enterprise Portal: Allegheny County Health Profiles." web page, undated. As of February 12, 2013: http://www.portal.state.pa.us/portal/server.pt?open=18&objID=1277942&mode=2

Cooper PJ, Murray L, Wilson A, Romaniuk H. "Controlled trial of the short- and long-term effect of psychological treatment of post-partum depression: (I. Impact on maternal mood)." *The British Journal of Psychiatry: The Journal of Mental Science,* 2003, 182: 412–419.

Cowen PS. "Crisis child care: An intervention for at-risk families." *Issues in Comprehensive Pediatric Nursing,* 1998, 21(3): 147–158.

Cummings EM, Schermerhorn AC, Keller PS, Davies PT. "Parental depressive symptoms, children's representations of family relationships, and child adjustment." *Social Development,* 2008, 17(2): 278–305.

Cutler, CB, Legano LA, Dreyer BP, Fierman AH, Berkule SB, Lusskin SI, Tomopoulos S, Roth M, Mendelsohn AL. "Screening for maternal depression in a low education population using a two item questionnaire." *Archives of Women's Mental Health,* 2007, 10(6): 277–283.

Davies PT, Winter MA, Cicchetti, D. "The implications of emotional security theory for understanding and treating childhood psychopathology." *Development and Psychopathology,* 2006, 8: 707–735.

Davis L, Edwards H, Mohay H, Wollin J. "The impact of very premature birth on the psychological health of mothers." *Early Human Development,* 2003, 73(1): 61–70.

Dennis CL, Hodnett E, Kenton L, Weston J, Zupancic J, Stewart DE, Kiss A. "Effect of peer support on prevention of postnatal depression among high risk women: Multisite randomised controlled trial." *British Medical Journal,* 2009, 33: a3064.

Devall EL. "Positive parenting for high-risk families." *Family and Consumer Sciences Research Journal,* 2004, 96(4): 7.

Diego MA, Field T, Hernandez-Reif M. "Prepartum, postpartum and chronic depression effects on neonatal behavior." *Infant Behavioral Development,* 2005, 28(5): 155–164.

Dietrich AWJ, Ciotti M, Schulkin J, Stotland N, Rost K, Cornell, J. "Depression care attitudes and practices of newer obstetrician-gynecologists: A national survey." *American Journal of Obstetrics and Gynecology,* 2003, 189(1): 267–273.

Dolezol S, Butterfield P. *How to Read Your Baby.* Denver, Colo.: Partners in Parenting Education, 1994.

Downey G, Coyne JC. "Children of depressed parents: An integrative review." *Psychological Bulletin,* 1990, 108(1): 50–76.

Dubowitz H, Feigelman S, Lane W, Prescott L, Blackman K, Grube L, Meyer W, Tracy JK. "Screening for depression in an urban pediatric primary care clinic." *Pediatrics,* 2007, 119(3): 435–443.

Elgar FJ, Mills RSL, McGrath PJ, Waschbusch DA, Brownridge DA. "Maternal and paternal depressive symptoms and child maladjustment: The mediating role of parental behavior." *Journal of Abnormal Child Psychology,* 2007, 35(6): 943–955.

Field TM. "Infants of depressed mothers." In *Stress, Coping, and Depression.* Johnson SL (ed.). Mahwah, N.J.: L. Erlbaum Associates, 2000, 3–23.

Flynn HA, Sexton M, Ratliff S, Porter K, Zivin K. "Comparative performance of the Edinburgh Postnatal Depression Scale and the Patient Health Questionnaire-9 in pregnant and postpartum women seeking psychiatric services." *Psychiatry Research,* 2011, 187(1–2): 130–134.

Garcia EFY, LaCaze C, Ratanasen M. "Continuous quality improvement for postpartum depression screening and referral." *Pediatrics International,* 2011, 53(2): 277–279.

Gaynes BN, Gavin N, Meltzer-Brody S, Lohr KN, Swinson T, Gartlehner G, Miller WC. *Perinatal Depression: Prevalence, Screening Accuracy, and Screening Outcomes.* Rockville, Md.: Agency for Healthcare Research and Quality, 2005. 1–8.

Goodman JH, Tyer-Viola L. "Detection, Treatment, and Referral of Perinatal Depression and Anxiety by Obstetrical Providers." *Journal of Women's Health,* 2010, 19(3): 477–490.

Goodman SH, Gotlib IH. "Risk for psychopathology in the children of depressed mothers: A developmental model for understanding mechanisms of transmission." *Psychological Review,* 1999, 106(3): 458–490.

Gordon TE, Cardone IA, Kim JJ, Gordon SM, Silver RK. "Universal perinatal depression screening in an Academic Medical Center." *Obstetrics and Gynecology,* 2006, 107(2): 342–347.

Gostin LO, Boufford JI, Martinez RM. "The future of the public's health: Vision, values, and strategies." *Health Affairs,* 2004, 23(4): 96–107.

Grace SL, Evindar A, Stewart DE. "The effect of postpartum depression on child cognitive development and behavior: A review and critical analysis of the literature." *Archives of Women's Mental Health,* 2003, 6(4): 263–274.

Heneghan AM, Morton S, DeLeone NL. "Paediatricians' attitudes about discussing maternal depression during a paediatric primary care visit." *Child: Care, Health and Development,* 2007, 33(3): 333–339.

Heneghan AM, Silver EJ, Bauman LJ, Stein RE. "Do pediatricians recognize mothers with depressive symptoms?" *Pediatrics,* 2000, 106(6): 1367–1373.

Hill LD, Greenberg BD, Holzman GB, Schulkin J. "Obstetrician-gynecologists' attitudes towards premenstrual dysphoric disorder and major depressive disorder." *Journal of Psychosomatic Obstetrics and Gynaecology,* 2001, 22(4): 241–250.

Howard KI, Kopta SM, Krause MS, Orlinsky DE. "The dose-effect relationship in psychotherapy." *American Psychologist,* 1986, 41(2): 159–164.

Ingram J, Taylor J. "Predictors of postnatal depression: Using an antenatal needs assessment discussion tool." *Journal of Reproductive and Infant Psychology,* 2007, 25(3): 210–222.

Institute for Healthcare Improvement. *The Breakthrough Series: IHI's Collaborative Model for Achieving Breakthrough Improvment.* Boston: Institute for Healthcare Improvement, 2003.

Institute of Medicine. *Crossing the Quality Chasm: A New Health System for the 21st Century.* Washington, D.C.: National Academy Press, 2001.

Institute of Medicine. *Improving the Quality of Health Care for Mental and Substance-Use Conditions.* Washington, D.C.: National Academies Press, 2006.

Institute of Medicine. *Preterm Birth: Causes, Consequences and Prevention.* Washington, D.C.: National Academies Press, 2007.

Kahn RS, Wise PH, Finkelstein JA, Bernstein HH, Lowe JA, Homer CJ. " The scope of unmet maternal health needs in pediatric settings." *Pediatrics,* 1999, 103(3): 576–581.

Kelly J, Zuckerman T, Sandoval D, Buehlman K. *Promoting First Relationships: A Curriculum for Service Providers to Help Parents and Other Caregivers Meet the Social and Emotional Needs of Young Children.* Seattle, Wash: NCAST Publications, 2003.

Kessler RC, McGonagle KA, Zhao S, Nelson CB, Hughes M, Eshleman S, Wittchen HU, Kendler KS. "Lifetime and 12-month prevalence of DSM-III-R psychiatric disorders in the United States: Results from the National Comorbidity Survey." *Archives of General Psychiatry,* 1994, 51(1): 8–19.

Keyser DJ, Beckjord EB, Firth R, Frith S, Lovejoy SL, Pillai S, Schultz D, Pincus HA. *Building Bridges: Lessons from a Pittsburgh Partnership to Strengthen Systems of Care for Maternal Depression.* Santa Monica, Calif.: RAND Corporation, MG-834, 2010. As of February 12, 2013: http://www.rand.org/pubs/monographs/MG973.html

Keyser DJ, Pincus HA, Thomas SB, Castle N, Dembosky J, Frith R, Greenberg M, Pollacj NK, Reis EC, Sansing VV, Scholle S. "Mobilizing a region to redesign a local system of care: Lessons from a community-based learning collaborative." *Family Community Health,* 2010, 3: 216–227.

Knitzer J, Theberge S, Johnson K. *Reducing Maternal Depression and Its Impact on Young Children: Toward a Responsive Early Childhood Policy Framework.* New York, N.Y.: Columbia University, Mailman School of Public Health, 2008.

Kroenke K., Spitzer, RL. "The PHQ-9: A New Depression Diagnostic and Severity Measure." *Psychiatric Annals,* 2002, 32(9).

Kroenke K., Spitzer RL, Williams JB. "The Patient Health Questionnaire-2: Validity of a two-item depression screener." *Medical Care,* 2003, 41: 1284–1292.

Kroenke K, Spitzer RL, Williams JB, Lowe B, "The Patient Health Questionnaire Somatic, Anxiety, and Depressive Symptom Scales: A systematic review." *General Hospital Psychiatry,* 2010, 32(4): 345–359.

Kuosmanen L, Vuorilehto M, Kumpuniemi S, Melartin T. "Post-natal depression screening and treatment in maternity and child health clinics." *Journal of Psychiatric and Mental Health Nursing,* 2010, 17(6): 554–557.

Lanzi RG, Pascoe JM, Keltner B, Ramey SL. "Correlates of maternal depressive symptoms in a national Head Start program sample." *Archives of Pediatrics and Adolescent Medicine,* 1999, 153(8): 801.

LaPerriere A, Ironson GH, Antoni MH, Pomm H, Jones D, Ishii M, et al. "Decreased depression up to one year following CBSM+ intervention in depressed women with AIDS: The smart/EST women's project." *Journal of Health Psychology,* 2005. 10, 223–231.

Lara MA, Navarro C, Rubi NA, Mondragon L. "Outcome results of two levels of intervention in low-income women with depressive symptoms." *The American Journal of Orthopsychiatry,* 2003, 73(1): 35–43.

LaRocco-Cockburn A, Melville J, Bell M, Katon W. "Depression screening attitudes and practices among obstetrician-gynecologists." *Obstetrics and Gynecology,* 2003, 101(5) Pt 1: 892–898.

Lillas C, Turnbull J. *Infant/Child Mental Health, Early Intervention, and Relationship-Based Therapies: A Neurorelational Framework for Interdisciplinary Practice.* New York: W. W. Norton & Co., Inc., 2009.

Lim JH, Wood BL, Miller BD. "Maternal depression and parenting in relation to child internalizing symptoms and asthma disease activity." *Journal of Family Psychology,* 2008, 22(2): 264–273.

Lipman EL, Boyle MH. "Social support and education groups for single mothers: A randomized controlled trial of a community-based program." *Canadian Medical Association Journal,* 2005, 173(12): 1451–1456.

Lovejoy MC, Graczyk PA, O'Hare E, Neuman G. "Maternal depression and parenting behavior: A meta-analytic review." *Clinical Psychology Review,* 2000, 20(5): 561–592.

MacArthur Initiative on Depression and Primary Care, "Patient Health Questionnaire PHQ-9 for Depression: Using PHQ-9 Diagnosis and Score for Initial Treatment Selection." web page, undated. As of February 12, 2013:
http://www.depression-primarycare.org

Marcus SM, Flynn HA, Blow FC, Barry KL. "Depressive symptoms among pregnant women screened in obstetrics settings." *Journal of Women's Health,* 2003, 12(4): 373–380.

Miller L, Gur M, Shanok A, Weissman M. "Interpersonal psychotherapy with pregnant adolescents: Two pilot studies." *Journal of Child Psychology and Psychiatry, and Allied Disciplines,* 2008, 49(7): 733–742.

Miller L, Shade M, Vasireddy V. "Beyond screening: Assessment of perinatal depression in a perinatal care setting." *Archives of Women's Mental Health,* 2009, 12(5): 329–334.

Miranda J, Chung JY, Green BL, Krupnick J, Siddique J, Revicki DA, Belin T. "Treating Depression in Predominantly Low-Income Young Minority Women: A Randomized Controlled Trial," *Journal of the American Medical Association,* 2003, 290(1): 57–65.

Miranda J, Green BL. "The need for mental health services research focusing on poor young women." *Journal of Mental Health Policy and Economics,* 1999, 2(2): 73–80.

Moore GA, Cohn JF, Campbell SB. "Infant affective responses to mother's still face at 6 months differentially predict externalizing and internalizing behaviors at 18 months." *Developmental Psychology,* 2001, 37(5): 706–714.

Mora PA, Bennett IM, Elo IT, Mathew L, Coyne JC, Culhane JF. "Distinct trajectories of perinatal depressive symptomatology: Evidence from growth mixture modeling." *American Journal of Epidemiology,* 2009, 169(1): 24–32.

Murray L, Cooper PJ, eds. *Postpartum Depression and Child Development.* New York, N.Y.: Guilford Press, 1997.

Murray L, Cooper PJ, Wilson A, Romaniuk H. "Controlled trial of the short- and long-term effect of psychological treatment of post-partum depression: (2. Impact on the mother-child relationship and child outcome)." *The British Journal of Psychiatry,* 2003, 182: 420–427.

Narrow WE. "One year prevalence of depressive disorders among adults 18 and over in the U.S.: NIMH ECA prospective data." Population estimates based on U.S. Census estimated residential population age 18 and over on July 1, 1998. Unpublished table.

National Center for Health Statistics. *National Vital Statistics Reports,* 2012, 61(6).

National Research Council and Institute of Medicine. *Depression in Parents, Parenting, and Children: Opportunities to Improve Identification, Treatment, and Prevention. Committee on Depression, Parenting Practices, and the Healthy Development of Children. Board on Children, Youth, and Families.* Division of Behavioral and Social Sciences and Education. Washington, D.C.: The National Academies Press, 2009.

O'Hara MW, Swain AM. "Rates and risk of postpartum depression: A meta-analysis." *International Review of Psychiatry,* 1996, 8: 37–54.

Olson AL, Kemper KJ, Kelleher KJ, Hammond CS, Zuckerman BS, Dietrich AJ. "Primary care pediatricians' roles and perceived responsibilities in the identification and management of maternal depression." *Pediatrics,* 2002, 110(6): 1169–1176.

OMAP—See Pennsylvania Office of Medical Assistance Programs.

Onunaku N. *Improving Maternal and Infant Mental Health: Focus on Maternal Depression.* Los Angeles, Calif.: National Center for Infant and Early Childhood Health Policy at UCLA, 2005.

Paulson JF, Dauber S, Leiferman JA. "Individual and combined effects of postpartum depression in mothers and fathers on parenting behavior," *Pediatrics,* 2006, 118(2): 659–668.

Peden AR. "A community-based depression prevention intervention with low-income single mothers." *Journal of the American Psychiatric Nurses Association,* 2005, 11(1): 18–25.

Pennsylvania Office of Medical Assistance Programs. *Statewide Performance Measures 2008–2009.*

Pennsylvania State Interagency Coordinating Council. *Early Intervention in Pennsylvania,* Annual report, 2010–2011. As of February 12, 2013:
http://pattan.net-website.s3.amazonaws.com/images/partner/2012/01/05/SICC%20Annual%20Rpt%20 2011_v5.pdf

Pepper CM, Maack DJ. "Course of depression." In *International Encyclopedia of Depression,* 2009.

Pincus HA, Houtsinger JK, Bachman J, Keyser D. "Depression in primary care: Bringing behavioral health care into the mainstream." *Health Affairs,* 2005, 4(1): 271–276.

Pleis JR, Ward BW, Lucas JW. Summary health statistics for U.S. adults: National Health Interview Survey, 2009. National Center for Health Statistics. *Vital Health Statistics,* 10(249). 2010.

Ramchandani P, Psychogiou L. "Paternal psychiatric disorders and children's psychosocial development." *The Lancet,* 2009, 374(9690): 646–653.

Ramos-Marcuse, F, Oberlander SE, Papas MA, McNary SW, Hurley KM, Black MM. "Stability of maternal depressive symptoms among urban, low-income, African American adolescent mothers." *Journal of Affective Disorders,* 2010, 122(1–2): 68–75.

Reitman D, Currier RO, Stickle TR. "A critical evaluation of the Parenting Stress Index-Short Form (PSI-SF) in a head start population." *Journal of Clinical Child and Adolescent Psychology,* 2002, 31(3): 384–392.

Robertson E, Grace S, Wallington T, Stewart DE. "Antenatal risk factors for postpartum depression: A synthesis of recent literature." *General Hospital Psychiatry,* 2004, 26(4): 289–295.

Ross LE, Dennis CL. "The prevalence of postpartum depression among women with substance use, an abuse history, or chronic illness: A systematic review." *Journal of Womens Health,* 2009, 18(4): 475–486.

Schultz D, Reynolds K, Sontag-Padilla L, Lovejoy SL, Firth R, Schake P, Hawk J, Killmeyer S, Troup E, Myers-Cepicka M, Perich M. *A Toolkit for Implementing Parental Depression Screening, Referral and Treatment Across Systems.* Santa Monica, Calif.: RAND Corporation, TL-102, 2012.

Segre LS, Brock RL, O'Hara MW, Gorman LL, Engeldinger J. "Disseminating perinatal depression screening as a public health initiative: A train-the-trainer approach." *Maternal and Child Health Journal,* 2011, 15(6): 814–821.

Sheeder J, Kabir K, Stafford B. "Screening for postpartum depression at well-child visits: Is once enough during the first six months of life?" *Pediatrics,* 2009, 123(6): E982–E988.

Seehusen DA, Baldwin LM, Runkle GP, Clark G. "Are family physicians appropriately screening for postpartum depression?" *The Journal of the American Board of Family Practice / American Board of Family Practice,* 2005, 18(2): 104–112.

Shaw DS, Connell A, Dishion TJ, Wilson MN, Gardner F. "Improvements in maternal depression as a mediator of intervention effects on early childhood problem behavior." *Development and Psychopathology,* 2009, 21(2): 417–439.

Shim RS, Baltrus P, Ye J, Rust G. "Prevalence, treatment, and control of depressive symptoms in the United States: Results from the National Health and Nutrition Examination Survey (NHANES), 2005–2008." *Journal of the American Board of Family Medicine,* 2011, 24(1): 33–38.

Siefert K, Bowman PJ, Heflin CM, Danziger S, Williams DR. "Social and environmental predictors of maternal depression in current and recent welfare recipients." *American Journal of Orthopsychiatry,* 2000, 70(4): 510–522.

Singer G. "Meta-analysis of comparative studies of depression in mothers of children with and without developmental disabilities." *Information,* 2006, 111(3): 155–169.

Singer LT, Salvator A, Guo S, Collin M, Lilien L, Baley J. "Maternal psychological distress and parenting stress after the birth of a very low-birth-weight infant." *Journal of American Medical Association,* 1999, 281(9): 799–805.

Sit DKY, Flint C, Svidergol D, White J, Wimer M, Bish B, Wisner K. "Best practices: An emerging best practice model for perinatal depression care." *Psychiatric Services,* 2009, 60(11): 1429–1431.

Skaer TL, Sclar DA, Robison LM, Galin RS. "Trends in the rate of depressive illness and use of antidepressant pharmacotherapy by ethnicity/race: An assessment of office-based visits in the United States, 1992–1997." *Clinical Therapy,* 2000, 22(12): 1575–1589.

Smith MV, Rosenheck RA, Cavaleri MA, Howell HB, Poschman K, Yonkers KA. "Screening for and detection of depression, panic disorder, and PTSD in public-sector obstetric clinics." *Psychiatric Services,* 2004, 55(4): 407–414.

Smith MV, Shao L, Howell H, Wang H, Poschman K, Yonkers KA. "Success of mental health referral among pregnant and postpartum women with psychiatric distress." *General Hospital Psychiatry,* 2009, 31(2): 155–162.

Sockol LE, Epperson CN, Barber JP. "A meta-analysis of treatments for perinatal depression." *Clinical Psychology Review,* 2011, 31(5): 839–849.

Sohr-Preston SL, Scaramella LV. "Implications of timing of maternal depressive symptoms for early cognitive and language development." *Clinical Child and Family Psychology Review,* 2006, 9(1): 65–83.

Sroufe LA, Egeland B, Carlson EA, and Collins WA. *The Development of the Person: The Minnesota Study of Risk and Adaptation from Birth to Adulthood.* New York: Guilford, 2005.

Thoppil J, Riutcel TL, Nalesnik SW. "Early intervention for perinatal depression." *American Journal of Obstetrics and Gynecology,* 2005, 192(5): 1446–1448.

Tronick E. *The Neurobehavioral and Social-Emotional Development of Infants and Children.* New York: WW Norton and Co., 2007.

U.S. Department of Agriculture. *The Consumer Data and Information Program Sowing the Seeds of Research.* Economic Research Service, 2009. As of February 13, 2012: http://www.ers.usda.gov/publications/ap-administrative-publication/ap-041.aspx

U.S. Department of Health and Human Services, Office of Women's Health. "Depression during and after pregnancy." Web page, last updated March 6, 2009. As of February 13, 2013: http://www.womenshealth.gov/publications/our-publications/fact-sheet/depression-pregnancy.html

van der Waerden JE, Hoefnagels C, Hosman CM. "Psychosocial preventive interventions to reduce depressive symptoms in low-SES women at risk: A meta-analysis." *Journal of Affective Disorders,* 2011, 128(1–2): 10–23.

Vesga-López O, Blanco C, Keyes K, Olfson M, Grant BF, Hasin DS. "Psychiatric disorders in pregnant and postpartum women in the United States." *Archive of General Psychiatry,* 2008, 65(7): 805–815.

Wagner EH. "Chronic disease management: What will it take to improve care for chronic illness?" *Effective Clinical Practices,* 1998, 1(1): 2–4.

Wagner EH, Austin BT, Davis C, Hindmarsh M, Schaefer J, Bonomi A. "Improving chronic illness care: Translating evidence into action." *Health Affairs,* 2001, 20(6): 64–78.

Wang PS, Berglund P, Kessler RC. "Recent care of common mental disorders in the United States: Prevalence and conformance with evidence-based recommendations." *Journal of General Internal Medicine,* 2000, 15(5): 284–292.

Weissman MM. "Remissions in Maternal Depression and Child Psychopathology: A STAR*D-Child Report." *Journal of the American Medical Association,* 2006, 295(12): 1389–1398.

Whitaker RC, Orzol SM, Kahn RS. "Maternal mental health, substance use, and domestic violence in the year after delivery and subsequent behavior problems in children at age 3 years." *Archive of General Psychiatry,* 2006, 63(5): 551–560.

Wiggins M, Oakley A, Roberts I, Turner H, Rajan L, Austerberry H, Mujica R, Mugford M, Barker M. "Postnatal support for mothers living in disadvantaged inner city areas: A randomised controlled trial." *Journal of Epidemiology and Community Health,* 2005, 59(4): 288–295.

Wilen JM, Mounts KO. "Women with depression—'You can't tell by looking'™." *Journal of Maternal and Child Health,* 2006, 10(suppl 1): 183–187.

Witt WP, Keller A, Gottlieb C, Litzelman K, Hampton J, Maguire J, Hagen EW. "Access to adequate outpatient depression care for mothers in the USA: A nationally representative population-based study." *Journal of Behavioral Health Services and Research,* 2009, PMID 19838806.

Yonkers KA, Smith MV, Lin H, Howell HB, Shao L, and Rosenheck RA. "Depression screening of perinatal women: An evaluation of the Healthy Start depression initiative." *Psychiatric Services,* 2009, 60: 322–328.

Young AS, Klap R, Sherbourne CD, Wells KB. "The quality of care for depressive and anxiety disorders in the United States." *Archive of General Psychiatry,* 2001 58(1): 55–61.